KETO DESSERT COOKBOOK
THE COMPLETE GUIDE

200 SWEET, TASTY AND LOW-CHOLESTEROL RECIPES
PERFECT FOR ANY OCCASION. BROWNIES, BARS, CAKES,
COOKIES, MOUSSE, KETOGENIC BOMBS AND MUCH MORE!

ANNA MOORE

TABLE OF CONTENTS

INTRODUCTION

Keto is an effective diet for weight loss. It has worked for many people in the past. It can be difficult to maintain, but is a great way to reduce your carb intake.

In addition to helping with weight loss, this diet can improve your health in many ways. It inhibits the effects of many chronic diseases such as diabetes, cancer, heart·disease, and Alzheimer's. It also helps to reduce inflammation in the body and increase metabolism - which both help with numerous diseases including diabetes.

Because many people choose to make low carb their way of life, there has been an increasing demand for low carb products. Our goal is to provide you with the finest products for your low carb lifestyle at an affordable price. We hope that you enjoy our products and that they help you toward your weight loss goals!

The keto diet is a low-carb eating plan. It's one of the most effective ways to lose weight and increase your metabolism. The keto diet limits both carbs and protein, allowing you to eat as much fat as you want. This is often called the "fat-burning" diet, and it's a popular way for people to improve their health and lose weight.

The keto diet also has many other benefits and is often used to treat medical conditions like epilepsy. It's popular at low carb conventions, where it's referred to as "ketogenic eating." Whether keto eating is right for you depends on your goals.

The keto diet is a high-fat, moderate-protein, and low-carbohydrate diet that forces your body to burn stored fat instead of carbs. The goal of the keto diet is to lose weight by starving the body of carbohydrates.

There are many diets out there. The keto diet was designed to help you lose weight by severely restricting carbs from your diet. On the keto diet, you eat animal proteins and fats in unlimited quantities, but you can't eat any fruits or vegetables because they're full of carbs. As a result, it's a high-fat, moderate protein diet.

How does it work?

Ketogenic diets are often prescribed for epilepsy and other diseases, but some people find that using a keto baking cookbook can help them eat healthier and lose weight.

When you think about how a diet works, you typically think about the foods that you eat. In fact, the type of food that you eat is the key to a ketogenic diet. You want to make sure that the foods that you eat are high in fat and very low in carbohydrates. This is what makes a keto diet so effective at helping people lose weight quickly.

The keto diet restricts many of the foods that most people eat in a regular diet. However, by following a cookbook full of delicious recipes, you can still enjoy some of your favorite foods.

If you're thinking about starting a keto diet, consider buying a keto baking cookbook from our website to help you enjoy your diet even more. It's one way that you can get started and start seeing results almost immediately!

CAKE RECIPES

1. MOIST AND DELICIOUS SPICE CAKE

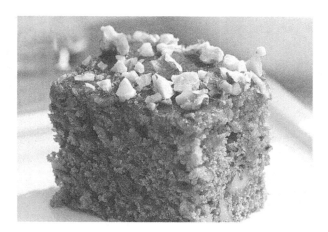

Preparation Time: 10 minutes - Cooking Time: 50 minutes - Servings: 10

Ingredients:

- 2 eggs - 2 cups almond flour - ½ tsp vanilla extract
- 1/3 cup water - 1/3 cup coconut oil, melted - ¼ tsp ground cloves
- 3 Tbsp. walnuts, chopped - ½ tsp ground ginger - 1 tsp ground cinnamon
- 2 tsp baking powder - ½ cup erythritol - Pinch of salt

Directions:

1. Spray a 7-inch cake pan with cooking spray and set aside.
2. Pour one cup of water into the Instant Pot and place a trivet in the pot.
3. In a large bowl, mix together almond flour, cloves, ginger, cinnamon, baking powder, erythritol, and salt.
4. Stir in the eggs, vanilla, water, and coconut oil until well mix.
5. Pour batter into the prepared cake pan and sprinkle with chopped walnuts.
6. Cover cake pan with aluminum foil and place it on top of trivet in the Instant Pot.
7. Seal pot with lid and cook on manual mode for 40 minutes.
8. When finished, allow pressure to release naturally for 10 minutes, and then release using the quick release method. Open the lid.
9. Remove cake pan from pot carefully and let it cool completely. Slice and serve.

Nutrition: Calories 220 Fat 20.8 g Carbs 5.9 g Sugar 0.9 g Protein 6.5 g Cholesterol 33 mg

2. CARROT CAKE

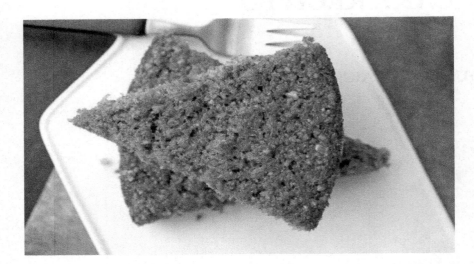

Preparation Time: 10 minutes - Cooking Time: 45 minutes - Servings: 8

Ingredients:

- 4 eggs - 1 cup pecans, chopped - 2¼ cups carrots, grated
- ¼ tsp nutmeg - 1 Tbsp. cinnamon - 1 Tbsp. baking powder
- 1 cup almond flour - 1½ cups coconut flour - 1 tsp vanilla extract
- 3/4 cup coconut oil, melted - ½ cup stevia Pinch of salt

Directions:

1. Spray a 7-inch cake pan with cooking spray and set aside.
2. Pour two cups of water into the Instant Pot and place a trivet in the pot.
3. In a mixing bowl, mix together sweetener, vanilla, and coconut oil.
4. Add eggs and stir well to combine.
5. Add coconut flour, nutmeg, cinnamon, baking powder, almond flour, and salt and stir to combine.
6. Add grated carrots and pecans and stir well. Pour batter into the prepared cake pan.
7. Cover cake pan with aluminum foil and place on top of the trivet.
8. Seal pot with lid and cook on steam mode for 45 minutes.
9. When finished, release pressure using the quick release method and then open the lid.
10. Remove cake from the pot and let it cool completely.
11. Slice and serve.

Nutrition: Calories 412 Fat 40.1 g Carbs 11.4 g Sugar 3 g Protein 7.9 g Cholesterol 82 mg

3. CHOCOLATE CAKE

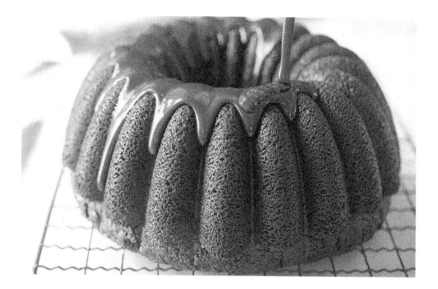

Preparation Time: 10 minutes - Cooking Time: 35 minutes - Servings: 8

Ingredients:

- 3 eggs - ¼ cup black coffee - ½ stick (2 oz.) butter
- 1 tsp baking powder - 1/3 cup erythritol - 1/3 cup cocoa powder
- ¼ cup coconut flour - ¼ cup flaxseed meal
- ½ cup almond flour - Pinch of salt

Directions:

1. Spray a cake pan with cooking spray and set aside.
2. Pour one cup of water into the Instant Pot and place a trivet in the pot.
3. In a large bowl, mix together almond flour, sweetener, cocoa powder, flax seed meal, and coconut flour.
4. Add remaining ingredients and stir until well combined.
5. Pour batter into the prepared cake pan and cover the pan with aluminum foil.
6. Place the cake pan on top of the trivet.
7. Seal pot with lid and cook on manual mode for 35 minutes.
8. When finished, allow pressure to release naturally for 10 minutes, then release using the quick released method. Open the lid.
9. Remove cake from the pot and let it cool completely.
10. Serve and enjoy.

Nutrition: Calories 143 Fat 12.5 g Carbs 5.1 g Sugar 0.5 g Protein 5 g Cholesterol 77 mg

4. FUDGY CHOCOLATE CAKE

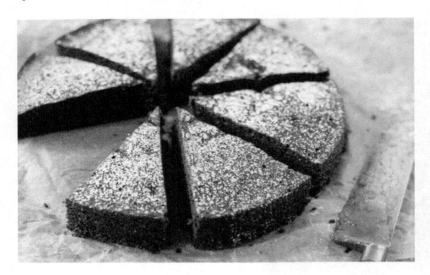

Preparation Time: 10 minutes - Cooking Time: 50 minutes - Servings: 8

Ingredients:

- 2 eggs, lightly beaten - 1 tsp vanilla extract - 1 Tbsp. coconut sugar
- ½ tsp baking soda - 1 cup almond flour - 2 Tbsp. coconut oil, melted
- ¼ cup unsweetened almond milk - 1 cup unsweetened chocolate chips - Pinch of salt

Directions:

1. Spray a 6-inch cake pan with cooking spray and set aside.
2. Pour two cups of water into the Instant Pot and place a trivet in the pot.
3. Add chocolate chips and almond milk to a saucepan and heat over low heat until chocolate has melted. Stir frequently. Once chocolate is melted, add coconut oil and stir to combine.
4. Remove saucepan from heat and let it cool completely.
5. In a large bowl, mix together all dry ingredients.
6. Add vanilla and eggs to the cool chocolate mixture and stir well.
7. Slowly add dry ingredients mixture and mix well.
8. Pour batter into the prepared cake pan and place cake pan on top of trivet in the pot.
9. Seal pot with lid and cook on manual mode for 40 minutes.
10. When finished, allow pressure to release naturally for 10 minutes, then release using the quick release method. Open the lid.
11. Remove cake from the pot and let it cool completely. Slice and serve

Nutrition: Calories 344 Fat 29.2 g Carbs 11.6 g Sugar 0.9 g Protein 8.6 g Cholesterol 41 mg

5. DELICIOUS COFFEE CAKE

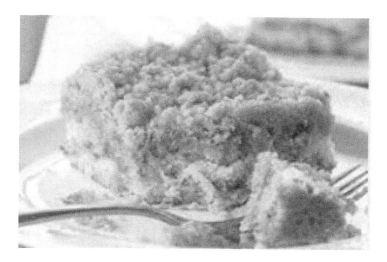

Preparation Time: 10 minutes - Cooking Time: 40 minutes - Servings: 8

Ingredients:

- 2 eggs - 1/4 tsp nutmeg - 1/2 tsp xanthan gum
- 1/2 tsp baking soda - 1 tbsp. baking powder
- 2 1/2 cups almond flour - 1 cup sour cream
- 1/2 cup Swerve - 1/2 cup butter, softened

For Topping:

- 1/4 cup butter, melted - 1 tsp cinnamon
- 2 tbsp. Swerve - 1 cup almond flour
- 1/4 cup pecans, chopped - Pinch of salt

Directions:

1. Preheat the oven to 350 F. Grease 9*9 cake pan and set aside.
2. In a mixing bowl, beat butter and sweetener until smooth. Add eggs and beat well.
3. Add sour cream and mix well. Add nutmeg, xanthan gum, baking soda, baking powder, and almond flour and blend well.
4. In a separate bowl, mix together all topping ingredients and set aside.
5. Pour cake batter into the prepared cake pan and sprinkle with topping mixture.
6. Bake cake for 35-40 minutes.
7. Allow the cake to cool completely. Slice and serve.

Nutrition: Calories 680 Fat 65.2 g Carbs 12.4 g Sugar 2 g Protein 2.8 g Cholesterol 84 mg

6. CHOCO PUDDING CAKE

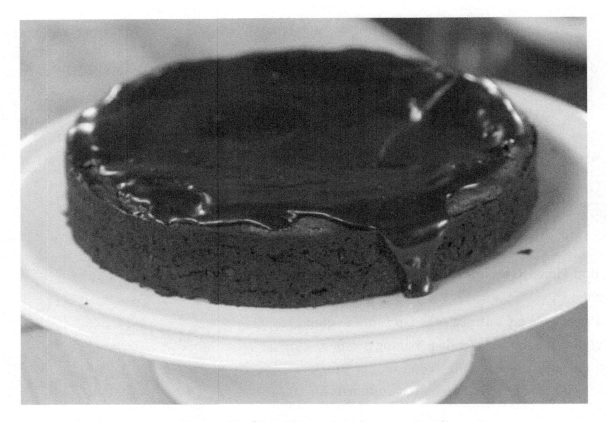

Preparation Time: 10 minutes - Cooking Time: 30 minutes - Servings: 6

Ingredients:

For cake:

- 3 eggs - 1 tsp baking powder
- 1 tsp vanilla extract - 2 Tbsp. erythritol
- 1 stick (4 oz) butter
- 3/4 cup unsweetened coconut milk
- 1/3 cup unsweetened cocoa powder
- ¼ cup coconut flour - 3/4 cup almond flour

For sauce:

- 1 cup hot water
- ¼ cup unsweetened cocoa powder
- 1 Tbsp. erythritol

Directions:

1. In a large bowl, mix together almond flour, cocoa powder, baking powder, sweetener, and coconut flour.
2. Add butter, coconut milk, and vanilla and mix until batter is smooth.
3. Add eggs and mix until well combined.
4. Spray a cake pan with cooking spray and pour batter into the pan.
5. In a separate bowl, whisk together all sauce ingredients.
6. Pour chocolate sauce over cake batter.
7. Cover cake pan with aluminum foil.
8. Pour two cups of water into the Instant Pot and place a trivet in the pot.
9. Place cake pan on top of the trivet in the pot.
10. Seal pot with lid and cook on high pressure for 30 minutes.
11. When finished, release pressure using the quick release method and open the lid carefully.
12. Remove cake from the pot and let it cool completely.
13. Slice and serve.

Nutrition: Calories 364 Fat 34.2 g Carbs 16.1 g Sugar 2.1 g Protein 10.2 g Cholesterol 122 mg

7. DELICIOUS ITALIAN CAKE

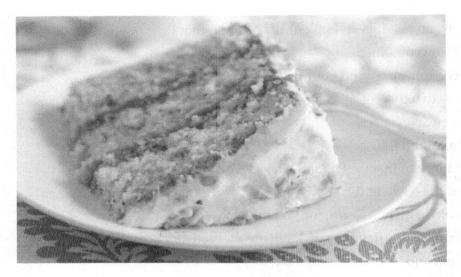

Preparation Time: 10 minutes - Cooking Time: 55 minutes - Servings: 12

Ingredients:

For cake:

- 5 eggs
- 2½ cups almond flour
- 1 tsp baking powder
- 1 cup unsweetened coconut flakes
- 2 tsp vanilla extract
- 2 cups Swerve confectioners' sugar
- 1 cup butter
- 1 tsp baking soda
- 1 cup sour cream

For frosting:

- 1 cup unsweetened coconut flakes
- ½ cup walnuts, chopped
- 2 Tbsp. unsweetened almond milk
- 2 cups Swerve confectioners' sugar
- 1 tsp vanilla extract
- ½ cup butter - 8 oz. cream cheese

Directions:

1. Pour one cup of water into the Instant Pot and place a trivet in the pot.
2. Spray a 7-inch cake pan with cooking spray and set aside.
3. In a small bowl, mix together sour cream and baking soda and set aside.
4. In a large bowl, whisk together 1 cup butter and the sweetener until fluffy.
5. Mix in the eggs, almond flour, baking powder, 1 cup coconut flakes, 2 tsp vanilla, and the sour cream mixture.
6. Pour batter in the prepared cake pan. Cover pan with aluminum foil.
7. Place cake pan on top of the trivet in the Instant Pot.
8. Seal pot with lid and cook on manual mode for 35 minutes.
9. When finished, allow pressure to release naturally for 20 minutes, and then release using the quick release method. Open the lid.
10. Remove cake from the pot and let it cool completely.
11. For frosting: In a mixing bowl, beat together ½ cup butter,
12. Swerve, cream cheese, and vanilla until fluffy.
13. Add almond milk, walnuts, and coconut flakes and stir well.
14. Spread frosting on top of the cake.
15. Slice and serve.

Nutrition: Calories 591 Fat 57.6 g Carbs 11.3 g Sugar 1.9 g Protein 11.9 g Cholesterol 158 mg

8. CLASSIC POUND CAKE

Preparation Time: 10 minutes - Cooking Time: 55 minutes - Servings: 10

Ingredients:

- 4 eggs - 1/2 cup sour cream - 1 tsp vanilla - 1 cup monk fruit sweetener - 1/4 cup butter
- 1/4 cup cream cheese - 1 tsp baking powder - 1 tbsp. coconut flour - 1 cup almond flour

Directions:

1. Preheat the oven to 350 F. Grease 9-inch cake pan and set aside.
2. In a mixing bowl, mix together almond flour, baking powder, and coconut flour.
3. In a separate bowl, add cream cheese and butter and microwave for 30 seconds.
4. Stir well and microwave for 30 seconds more. Stir in sour cream, vanilla, and sweetener.
5. Mix to combine. Pour cream cheese mixture into the almond flour mixture and stir until well combined.
6. Add eggs in batter one by one and stir until well combined.
7. Pour batter into the prepared cake pan. Bake cake for 55 minutes.
8. Allow the cake to cool completely. Slice and serve.

Nutrition: Calories 211 Fat 17 g Carbohydrates 8.3 g Sugar 5.5 g Protein 3.2 g Cholesterol 89 mg

9. MOIST CARROT CAKE

Preparation Time: 10 minutes - Cooking Time: 30 minutes - Servings: 10

Ingredients:

- 4 eggs - 2 cups grated carrots - 2 tsp baking powder - 1/2 tsp xanthan gum
- 1/2 tsp nutmeg - 2 tsp cinnamon - 2 tbsp. coconut flour - 2 cups almond flour
- 2 tsp vanilla - 3/4 cup Swerve - 3/4 cup butter - Pinch of salt

Directions:

1. Preheat the oven to 350 F. Grease cake pan and set aside.
2. In a mixing bowl, beat butter and sweetener until light and fluffy. Add vanilla and eggs one by one and beat well.
3. In a separate bowl, mix together almond flour, baking powder, xanthan gum, nutmeg, cinnamon, coconut flour, and salt.
4. Add almond flour mixture into the butter and egg mixture and stir until just combined.
5. Add grated carrots and stir well.
6. Pour batter into the prepared cake pan and bake for 25-30 minutes.
7. Allow the cake to cool completely. Slice and serve.

Nutrition: Calories 312 Fat 28 g Carbohydrates 8.3 g Sugar 2.3 g Protein 2.8 g Cholesterol 102 mg

10. GOOEY & RICH BUTTER CAKE

Preparation Time: 10 minutes - Cooking Time: 45 minutes - Servings: 15

Ingredients:

For crust:

- 1 egg - 2 cups almond flour - 1/2 tsp vanilla - 1/2 cup butter, melted
- 2 tsp baking powder - 2 tbsp. whey protein powder - 1/2 cup Swerve - Pinch of salt

For filling:

- 2 eggs - 1/2 tsp vanilla - 3/4 cup Swerve
- 1/2 cup butter, softened - 8 oz. cream cheese, softened

Directions:

1. Preheat the oven to 325 F. Grease 9*13 cake pan and set aside. In a mixing bowl, mix together almond flour, baking powder, protein powder, sweetener, and salt.
2. Add egg, vanilla, and butter and stir until well combined. Pour almond flour mixture into the prepared pan and spread well and press down.
3. For filling: In a separate bowl, beat butter and cream cheese until smooth. Add sweetener and beat until combined. Add vanilla and eggs and beat until smooth.
4. Pour filling over crust and bake for 35-45 minutes. Allow the cake to cool completely. Slice and serve.

Nutrition: Calories 274 Fat 26.5 g Carbohydrates 3.7 g Sugar 0.7 g Protein 2.9 g Cholesterol 83 mg

11. LEMON POUND CAKE

Preparation Time: 10 minutes - Cooking Time: 60 minutes - Servings: 16

Ingredients:

- 6 eggs - 2 egg yolks - 2 tsp lemon extract - 1/3 cup erythritol - 2 cups almond flour
- 4 oz. cream cheese, softened - 1 cup butter, softened - 2 tsp xanthan gum

Directions:

1. Preheat the oven to 325 F. Grease 9*5 loaf pan and set aside.
2. In a mixing bowl, mix together almond flour and xanthan gum and set aside.
3. In a large bowl, beat cream cheese and butter until smooth.
4. Add sweetener and lemon extract and beat until the mixture becomes fluffy.
5. Add eggs and eggs yolk one by one and beat until well combined.
6. Add almond flour mixture and beat until just combined. Do not over mix.
7. Pour batter into the prepared loaf pan and bake for 60 minutes.
8. Allow the cake to cool completely. Slice and serve.

Nutrition: Calories 249 Fat 23.7 g Carbohydrates 3.2 g Sugar 0.7 g Protein 3 g Cholesterol 126 mg

12. NUTELLA MUG CAKE

Preparation Time: 10 minutes - Cooking Time: 1 minute - Servings: 1

Ingredients:

- 1 egg - 2 tbsp. Swerve - 1/2 tsp baking powder
- 1 tbsp. unsweetened cocoa powder
- 3 tbsp. hazelnut flour - 1 tbsp. butter, melted

Directions:

1. Add all ingredients into the microwave-safe mug and whisk until smooth.
2. Microwave for 60 seconds. Serve and enjoy.

Nutrition: Calories 325 Fat 29.4 g Carbohydrates 12 g Sugar 1.2 g Protein 9.7 g Cholesterol 194 mg

13. PERFECT PUMPKIN CRUMB CAKE

Preparation Time: 10 minutes - Cooking Time: 40 minutes - Servings: 16

Ingredients:

- 2 eggs - 1/2 tsp vanilla - 1/4 cup butter, melted - 1/2 cup pumpkin puree
- 3/4 tsp pumpkin pie spice - 2 tsp baking powder - 1/4 cup whey protein powder
- 1/3 cup coconut flour - 1/2 cup Swerve - 1 cup almond flour - Pinch of salt

For topping:

- 1 cup almond flour - 1/2 cup butter, melted - 1/2 tsp pumpkin pie spice
- 1/2 cup Swerve - 1/4 cup coconut flour - Pinch of salt

Directions:

1. Preheat the oven to 325 F. Grease 9*9-inch cake pan and set aside.
2. Add all topping ingredients into the medium bowl and mix until well combined and set aside.
3. In a large bowl, mix together almond flour, pumpkin pie spice, baking powder, protein powder, coconut flour, sweetener, and salt.
4. Stir in eggs, vanilla, butter, pumpkin puree until well combined.
5. Pour batter into the prepared cake pan and spread well.
6. Sprinkle topping mixture evenly on top of cake batter.
7. Bake cake for 35-40 minutes.
8. Allow the cake to cool completely. Slice and serve.

Nutrition: Calories 202 Fat 17.3 g Carbohydrates 6.5 g Sugar 1 g Protein 2.5 g Cholesterol 46 mg

14. CARROT CAKE WITH FROSTING

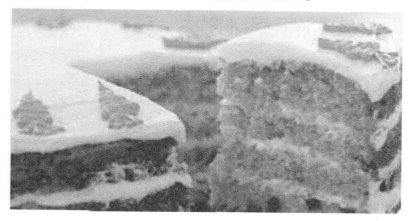

Preparation Time: 10 minutes - Cooking Time: 25 minutes - Servings: 12

Ingredients:

- 4 eggs - 1/2 cup grated carrot - 1/4 tsp ground allspice
- 1 1/2 tsp ground cinnamon - 1 tbsp. baking powder - 2 tbsp. coconut flour
- 1 1/2 cups almond flour - 1 tsp vanilla - 2 tbsp. almond milk
- 5 tbsp. butter, softened - 1/2 cup erythritol

For frosting:

- 4 oz. cream cheese, softened - 1/4 cup erythritol
- 1 tbsp. heavy cream - 1 tsp vanilla - 2 tbsp. butter, softened

Directions:

1. Preheat the oven to 350 F. Grease 9-inch cake pan and set aside.
2. In a large bowl, beat butter and sweetener until fluffy. Add eggs and beat well.
3. Add vanilla and almond milk and stir well.
4. Add spices, baking powder, coconut flour, and almond flour and beat until just combined.
5. Add grated carrot and fold well.
6. Pour batter into the prepared cake pan and bake for 20-25 minutes.
7. Once done remove from oven and set aside to cool completely.
8. For frosting: In a medium bowl, beat cream cheese and butter until smooth.
9. Add vanilla and sweetener and beat well.
10. Add heavy cream and stir well. Once the cake is cool then spread frosting on top.
11. Slice and serve.

Nutrition: Calories 224 Fat 20.2 g Carbohydrates 5.1 g Sugar 1.1 g Protein 2.9 g Cholesterol 85 mg

15. CHOCOLATE FLOURLESS CAKE

Preparation Time: 10 minutes - Cooking Time: 45 minutes - Servings: 16

Ingredients:

- 6 eggs - 1 tbsp. vanilla - 1/4 cup unsweetened cocoa powder - 5 oz. butter
- 2 tbsp. instant espresso powder - 1 cup erythritol -10 oz. dark chocolate chips

Directions:

1. Preheat the oven to 350 F. Grease 8-inch springform pan and set aside.
2. Add chocolate chips and butter in a bowl and melt in a double boiler. Stir well.
3. Add espresso powder and sweetener and sit well.
4. Remove bowl from heat and let it cool for 10 minutes.
5. Add vanilla, cocoa powder, and eggs into the melted chocolate mixture and beat using a hand mixer until smooth.
6. Pour batter into the prepared cake pan and bake for 45 minutes.
7. Allow the cake to cool completely. Slice and serve.

Nutrition: Calories 175 Fat 13.7 g Carbohydrates 12.8 g Sugar 9.7 g Protein 3.6 g Cholesterol 80mg

16. LIGHT & FLUFFY COFFEE CAKE

Preparation Time: 10 minutes - Cooking Time: 30 minutes - Servings: 12

Ingredients:

- 3 eggs - 1/2 cup macadamia nuts, chopped - 1/4 tsp ground allspice
- 1 tsp vanilla - 1 tsp baking powder - 1 tbsp. ground cinnamon
- 1/2 cup Swerve - 1/4 cup almond flour - 1/4 cup coconut flour
- 1/4 cup ground flax - 1/2 cup sour cream - 1/4 cup butter - Pinch of salt

Directions:

1. Preheat the oven to 350 F. Grease 8*8-inch cake pan and set aside.
2. In a medium bowl, whisk eggs. Add cream and butter and stir to combine.
3. In a separate bowl, mix together all dry ingredients.
4. Add dry ingredient mixture into the egg mixture and blend until well combined.
5. Pour batter into the prepared cake pan and bake for 30 minutes.
6. Allow the cake to cool completely. Slice and serve.

Nutrition: Calories 162 Fat 14.4 g Carbohydrates 5.2 g Sugar 0.7 g Protein 3.2 g Cholesterol 55 mg

17. MOIST COCONUT POUND CAKE

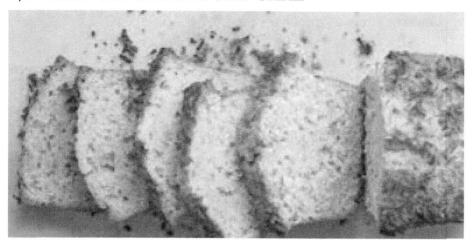

Preparation Time: 10 minutes - Cooking Time: 45 minutes - Servings: 8

Ingredients:

- 4 eggs
- 1 tsp vanilla
- 1/2 cup coconut yogurt
- 1/2 cup Swerve
- 4 tbsp. coconut oil
- 1 tsp baking powder
- 1 1/4 cups almond flour
- Pinch of salt

Directions:

1. Preheat the oven to 350 F.
2. Grease 8-inch loaf pan and set aside.
3. In a medium bowl, mix together almond flour, baking powder, and salt and set aside.
4. In a large mixing bowl, beat together sweetener and coconut oil until light.
5. Add eggs, vanilla, and coconut yogurt and beat until well combined.
6. Add almond flour mixture into the wet mixture and beat until just combined.
7. Pour batter into the prepared loaf pan and bake for 40-5 minutes.
8. Allow the cake to cool completely.
9. Slice and serve.

Nutrition: Calories 206 Fat 18.4 g Carbohydrates 4 g Sugar 0.9 g Protein 2.8 g Cholesterol 82 mg

18. SUPER EASY CHOCOLATE CAKE

Preparation Time: 10 minutes - Cooking Time: 25 minutes - Servings: 8

Ingredients:

- 5 eggs - 2/3 cup erythritol - 2/3 cup butter, melted - 9 oz. unsweetened dark chocolate
- 1 tsp baking powder - 1/2 cup almond flour - 1 tsp vanilla - Pinch of salt

Directions:

1. Preheat the oven to 350 F. Grease cake pan and set aside.
2. In a mixing bowl, mix together almond flour, baking powder, and salt and set aside.
3. Melt butter and chocolate together. Stir well and let it cool.
4. Transfer melted butter and chocolate mixture into the medium bowl.
5. Add eggs one by one and beat until smooth.
6. Add almond flour mixture, sweetener, and vanilla and blend well.
7. Pour batter into the prepared cake pan and bake for 20-25 minutes.
8. Allow the cake to cool completely.
9. Slice and serve.

Nutrition: Calories 384 Fat 39 g Carbohydrates 10 g Sugar 0.5 g Protein 8.3 g Cholesterol 143 mg

19. CREAM CHEESE POUND CAKE

Preparation Time: 10 minutes - Cooking Time: 40 minutes - Servings: 12

Ingredients:

- 4 eggs - 1 tsp vanilla - 4 tbsp. butter - 3.5 oz. cream cheese
- 1 tsp baking powder - 3/4 cup erythritol - 1 1/4 cups almond flour - Pinch of salt

Directions:

1. Preheat the oven to 350 F. Grease 8-inch loaf pan and set aside.
2. In a mixing bowl, mix together almond flour, baking powder, and salt and set aside.
3. In a large bowl, beat butter and sweetener until fluffy.
4. Add cream cheese and vanilla and mix well. Add eggs one by one and beat well.
5. Add almond flour mixture and blend until well combined.
6. Pour batter into the prepared loaf pan and bake for 30-40 minutes.
7. Allow the cake to cool completely. Slice and serve.

Nutrition: Calories 160 Fat 14.4 g Carbohydrates 2.7 g Sugar 0.6 g Protein 2.5 g Cholesterol 74 mg

20. MOIST VANILLA CAKE

Preparation Time: 10 minutes - Cooking Time: 40 minutes - Servings: 8

Ingredients:

- 6 egg whites - 1 tsp baking powder - 1/4 cup coconut flour
- 1 cup almond flour - 1/2 cup Swerve - 1/4 cup sour cream
- 1 tsp vanilla - 1/4 cup coconut oil, melted - Pinch of salt

Directions:

1. Preheat the oven to 350 F. Grease loaf pan and set aside.
2. In a mixing bowl, whisk together vanilla and coconut oil.
3. Add sour cream and whisk until combined.
4. Add sweetener and egg whites one by one and beat until combined.
5. Stir in flours, baking powder, and salt and blend until well combined.
6. Pour batter into the prepared loaf pan and bake for 30-40 minutes.
7. Allow the cake to cool completely. Slice and serve.

Nutrition: Calories 194 Fat 16.4 g Carbohydrates 5.5 g Sugar 1 g Protein 3.4 g Cholesterol 3 mg

21. PERFECT BLACKBERRY CAKE

Preparation Time: 10 minutes - Cooking Time: 60 minutes - Servings: 16

Ingredients:

For cake:

- 4 eggs - 1 tsp vanilla - 1/2 cup coconut milk - 1/3 cup coconut milk, melted
- 1/2 cup Swerve - 1 tsp baking powder - 1/4 cup coconut flour - 1 1/4 cups almond flour

For topping:

- 2 tbsp. coconut oil - 2 tbsp. Swerve - 1 cup almonds - 2 cups blackberries

Directions:

1. Preheat the oven to 350 F. Grease 8*8-inch cake pan and set aside.
2. For cake: In a medium bowl, mix together all dry ingredients. Add remaining cake ingredients and mix until well combined.
3. Pour batter into the prepared cake pan. Sprinkle blackberries on top.
4. Bake cake for 15 minutes. Meanwhile, add almond, swerve, and coconut oil into the food processor and process until wet crumb mixture form.
5. Sprinkle crumb mixture on top of the cake and bake a cake for 40-45 minutes more.
6. Allow the cake to cool completely. Slice and serve.

Nutrition: Calories 167 Fat 13.8 g Carbohydrates 6.8 g Sugar 2.1 g Protein 3.4 g Cholesterol 41 mg

22. PERFECT GINGERBREAD CAKE

Preparation Time: 10 minutes - Cooking Time: 45 minutes - Servings: 12

Ingredients:

- 4 eggs - 1/4 cup water - 1/4 tsp ground nutmeg - 1/8 tsp ground cloves
- 1 tsp ground cinnamon - 1 tsp ground ginger - 1 tsp baking powder
- 2 tbsp. psyllium husk powder - 3/4 cup almond flour - 1/4 cup coconut flour
- 1/2 cup Swerve - 1/2 cup butter - Pinch of salt

Directions:

1. Preheat the oven to 350 F. Grease 9-inch loaf pan and set aside.
2. In a large bowl, beat butter and sweetener until fluffy.
3. Add eggs one by one and beat until well combined.
4. In a separate bowl, mix together almond flour, cloves, nutmeg, cinnamon, ginger, baking powder, psyllium husk, coconut flour, and salt.
5. Add almond flour mixture into the egg mixture and blend until well combined.
6. Add water and stir until smooth.
7. Pour batter into the prepared loaf pan and bake for 45 minutes.
8. Allow the cake to cool completely. Slice and serve.

Nutrition: Calories 151 Fat 13.2 g Carbohydrates 4.6 g Sugar 0.6 g Protein 2.3 g Cholesterol 75 mg

23. CHOCOLATE ZUCCHINI CAKE

Preparation Time: 10 minutes - Cooking Time: 30 minutes - Servings: 16

Ingredients:

- 3 eggs - 3 tbsp. coconut milk - 3 tbsp. coconut oil, melted
- 1/4 cup shredded zucchini - 1/2 tsp baking powder - 1/4 tsp baking soda
- 1/2 cup Swerve - 1/4 cup unsweetened cocoa powder - 1/4 cup coconut flour

Directions:

1. Preheat the oven to 350 F. Grease 8*8-inch cake pan and set aside.
2. Add all ingredients into the blender and blend until a thick batter is a form.
3. Pour batter into the prepared pan and bake for 25-30 minutes.
4. Allow the cake to cool completely. Slice and serve.

Nutrition: Calories 51 Fat 4.5 g Carbohydrates 2.2 g Sugar 0.3 g Protein 1.6 g Cholesterol 31 mg

24. PERFECT ALMOND CRUMB CAKE

Preparation Time: 10 minutes - Cooking Time: 40 minutes - Servings: 16

Ingredients:

For cake:

- 4 eggs - 1 tsp baking powder - 1 cup almond flour - 1/2 cup coconut flour - 2 tbsp. butter
- 4 oz. half and half - 2 tsp vanilla - 1/3 cup Swerve - 2 oz. cream cheese, softened

For topping:

- 1 cup sliced almonds, toasted - 1 cup almond flour - 1/3 cup Swerve - 6 tbsp. butter, melted

Directions:

1. Preheat the oven to 350 F. Grease 8*8-inch cake pan and set aside.
2. Add all cake ingredients into the large mixing bowl and beat until well combined.
3. Pour batter into the prepared cake pan.
4. Mix together all topping ingredients and sprinkle on top of cake batter.
5. Bake cake for 40 minutes. Allow the cake to cool completely. Slice and serve.

Nutrition: Calories 230 Fat 19.9 g Carbohydrates 6.5 g Sugar 1.2 g Protein 3.7 g Cholesterol 63 mg

25. BLUEBERRY CAKE

Preparation Time: 10 minutes - Cooking Time: 40 minutes - Servings: 10

Ingredients:

For cake:

- 2 eggs - 1 1/2 tsp baking powder - 1/2 cup coconut flour
- 1 tsp vanilla - 1/2 cup butter, softened

For filling:

- 1 cup blueberries - 1/3 cup xylitol - 1 tsp vanilla - 3 eggs - 1 cup sour cream

Directions:

1. Preheat the oven to 350 F. Grease 8-inch spring-form pan and set aside.
2. In a mixing bowl, beat butter and sweetener until light.
3. Add vanilla and egg one by one and beat until well combined.
4. Mix together coconut flour and baking powder and add into the egg mixture and blend until well combined.
5. Pour batter into the prepared pan and set aside.
6. For filling: In a large bowl, whip sour cream, sweetener, vanilla, and eggs until creamy.
7. Pour over cake batter. Sprinkle blueberries evenly on top of cake batter.
8. Bake cake for 35-40 minutes. Allow the cake to cool completely. Slice and serve.

Nutrition: Calories 203 Fat 16.9 g Carbohydrates 9 g Sugar 1.8 g Protein 4.5 g Cholesterol 116 mg

26. BROWNIE MUG CAKE

Preparation Time: 10 minutes - Cooking Time: 2 minutes - Servings: 1

Ingredients:

- 1 egg - 1/2 tsp baking powder
- 1 tbsp. Swerve
- 1 tbsp. unsweetened chocolate chips
- 1 tbsp. unsweetened cocoa powder
- 1/4 cup almond flour
- 1 tbsp. butter, melted

Directions:

1. Add all ingredients into the microwave-safe mug and stir until well combined.
2. Place in microwave and microwave for 2 minutes.
3. Serve and enjoy.

Nutrition: Calories 355 Fat 30 g Carbohydrates 13.9 g Sugar 3.9 g Protein 7.6 g Cholesterol 164 mg

27. PEANUT BUTTER MUG CAKE

Preparation Time: 10 minutes - Cooking Time: 1 minute - Servings: 6

Ingredients:

- 3 tbsp. unsweetened chocolate chips
- 1/4 cup water - 1/2 tsp vanilla
- 2 eggs - 2 tsp baking powder
- 1/3 cup Swerve - 2/3 cup almond flour
- 1/4 cup butter - 1/3 cup peanut butter

Directions:

1. Melt butter and peanut butter in a microwave-safe bowl. Stir until smooth.
2. In a medium bowl, mix together almond flour, baking powder, and sweetener.
3. Stir in melted butter mixture, eggs, and vanilla.
4. Add water and stir until well combined. Add chocolate chips and stir well.
5. Divide mixture into the 6 ramekins and microwave for 1 minute.
6. Serve warm and enjoy.

Nutrition: Calories 257 Fat 22.4 g Carbohydrates 7.9 g Sugar 1.8 g Protein 8.4 g Cholesterol 75 mg

28. VANILLA MUG CAKE

Preparation Time: 10 minutes - Cooking Time: 1 minute - Servings: 1

Ingredients:

- 1 egg - 1/4 tsp baking powder - 1/4 tsp vanilla
- 1 tbsp. Swerve - 1 tbsp. coconut flour - 1 oz. cream cheese, softened

Directions:

1. In a small bowl, whisk egg, cream cheese, and vanilla for 2 minutes.
2. Add remaining ingredients and stir until well combined.
3. Pour mixture into the microwave-safe mug and microwave for 1 minute.
4. Serve warm and enjoy.

Nutrition: Calories 201 Fat 15 g Carbohydrates 8.8 g Sugar 0.5 g Protein 8.7 g Cholesterol 195 mg

29. CHOCO CHIP MUG CAKE

Preparation Time: 10 minutes - Cooking Time: 1 minute - Servings: 1

Ingredients:

- 1 egg, lightly beaten - 1/2 tsp baking powder - 2 tbsp. Swerve
- 2 tbsp. unsweetened chocolate chips - 2 tbsp. unsweetened cocoa powder
- 1/4 cup almond flour - 2 tbsp. butter, melted - Pinch of salt

Directions:

1. Add all ingredients into the microwave-safe mug and stir to combine.
2. Microwave for 1 minute.
3. Top with whipped cream and serve.

Nutrition: Calories 333 Fat 31.7 g Carbohydrates 10.5 g Sugar 1 g Protein 8 g Cholesterol 225 mg

30. SNICKERDOODLE MUG CAKE

Preparation Time: 10 minutes - Cooking Time: 1 minute - Servings: 1

Ingredients:

- 1 egg - 1/2 tsp cinnamon - 1/2 tsp vanilla - 1 tbsp. Swerve
- 1/2 tsp baking powder - 3 tbsp. almond flour - 1 tbsp. butter, melted

Directions:

1. Add all ingredients into the microwave-safe mug and whisk until smooth.
2. Microwave for 30 seconds to 1 minute. Serve and enjoy.

Nutrition: Calories 307 Fat 26 g Carbohydrates 9.2 g Sugar 0.6 g Protein 10 g Cholesterol 194 mg

31. PUMPKIN SPICE MUG CAKE

Preparation Time: 10 minutes - Cooking Time: 1 minute - Servings: 1

Ingredients:

- 1 egg, lightly beaten - 1/4 tsp nutmeg - 1/2 tsp cinnamon - 2 tsp pumpkin spice
- 1 tsp vanilla - 1 tsp baking powder - 2 tbsp. Swerve - 1 tbsp. coconut flour
- 2 tbsp. almond flour - 1 tbsp. sour cream - 1 tbsp. butter, melted

Directions:

1. Add all ingredients into the microwave-safe mug and whisk until smooth.
2. Microwave for 60 seconds. Serve and enjoy.

Nutrition: Calories 355 Fat 27.6 g Carbohydrates 18 g Sugar 2.3 g Protein 7.3 g Cholesterol 199 mg

32. SWEET & TANGY LEMON MUG CAKE

Preparation Time: 10 minutes - Cooking Time: 1 minute - Servings: 1

Ingredients:

- 1 egg - 1/2 tsp lemon rind - 1 tbsp. butter, melted - 2 tbsp. fresh lemon juice
- 1 tsp Swerve - 1/2 tsp baking powder - 1/4 cup almond flour

Directions:

1. Add all ingredients into the microwave-safe mug and whisk until smooth.
2. Microwave for 90 seconds. Serve and enjoy.

Nutrition: Calories 360 Fat 31.2 g Carbohydrates 9.4 g Sugar 2 g Protein 5.9 g Cholesterol 194 mg

33. MOIST CARROT MUG CAKE

Preparation Time: 10 minutes - Cooking Time: 5 minutes - Servings: 2

Ingredients:

- 1 egg - 1 tsp baking powder - 1 tsp pumpkin spice - 2 tsp cinnamon - 2 tbsp. erythritol
- 3/4 cup almond flour - 1 tbsp. heavy cream - 2 tbsp. butter, melted - 1/2 cup grated carrot

Directions:

1. In a medium bowl, mix together almond flour, sweetener, baking powder, pumpkin spice, and cinnamon.
2. In a separate bowl, whisk together heavy cream, butter, egg, and grated carrot.
3. Add almond flour mixture into the heavy cream mixture and mix until well combined.
4. Pour batter into the 2 ramekins and microwave for 5 minutes at 800W. Serve and enjoy.

Nutrition: Calories 451 Fat 39 g Carbohydrates 14.2 g Sugar 3.2 g Protein 3.4 g Cholesterol 123 mg

34. SUPER EASY BLUEBERRY MUG CAKE

Preparation Time: 10 minutes - Cooking Time: 1 minute - Servings: 1

Ingredients:

- 1 egg - 1 tbsp. blueberries - 2 tbsp. coconut flour - 1/4 tsp baking powder
- 2 tbsp. Swerve - 2 tbsp. fresh lemon juice - 1 tbsp. butter, melted

Directions:

1. Add all ingredients except blueberries into the microwave-safe mug and whisk until smooth.
2. Add blueberries and stir well. Microwave for 90 seconds. Serve and enjoy.

Nutrition: Calories 248 Fat 18.2 g Carbohydrates 14.8 g Sugar 2.8 g Protein 8g Cholesterol 194 mg

35. PUMPKIN COCONUT MUG CAKE

Preparation Time: 10 minutes - Cooking Time: 1 minute - Servings: 1

Ingredients:

- 1 egg - 1/4 tsp vanilla - 1 tbsp. Swerve - 2 tbsp. coconut oil, melted - 2 tbsp. pumpkin puree
- 1/2 tsp pumpkin pie spice - 1/4 tsp baking soda - 2 tbsp. coconut flour

Directions:

1. Add all ingredients into the microwave-safe mug and whisk until smooth.
2. Microwave for 60 seconds. Serve and enjoy.

Nutrition: Calories 379 Fat 33.8 g Carbohydrates 13.5 g Sugar 2.6 g Protein 8 g Cholesterol 164 mg

36. STRAWBERRY MUG CAKE

Preparation Time: 10 minutes - Cooking Time: 1 minute - Servings: 2

Ingredients:

- 1 egg, lightly beaten - 1/4 cup strawberries, chopped - 1 tsp vanilla
- 1/2 tsp baking soda - 1 tsp baking powder - 2 tbsp. Swerve - 1 tbsp. coconut flour
- 2 tbsp. almond flour - 1 tbsp. sour cream - 1 tbsp. butter, melted

Directions:

1. Grease 2 ramekins and set aside.
2. In a mixing bowl, whisk together egg, vanilla, baking soda, baking powder, sweetener, coconut flour, almond flour, and sour cream until well combined.
3. Divide strawberries into the two ramekins. Evenly pour batter between two ramekins.
4. Microwave for 90 seconds. Serve and enjoy.

Nutrition: Calories 174 Fat 13.5 g Carbohydrates 8.5 g Sugar 1.8 g Protein 3.6 g Cholesterol 99 mg

37. DELICIOUS BERRY CAKE

Preparation Time: 10 minutes - Cooking Time: 1 minute - Servings: 1

Ingredients:

- 1 egg - 5 frozen raspberries - 1/4 tsp baking powder - 1 tsp vanilla
- 1 tbsp. Swerve - 2 tbsp. coconut flour - 2 tbsp. cream cheese - 1 tbsp. butter, melted

Directions:

1. Add all ingredients except raspberries into the microwave-safe mug and whisk until smooth.
2. Add raspberries and stir well.
3. Microwave on high for 80 seconds.
4. Serve and enjoy.

Nutrition: Calories 323 Fat 24.9 g Carbohydrates 14.6 g Sugar 4g Protein 9.2 g Cholesterol 216 mg

38. VANILLA COCONUT CAKE

Preparation Time: 10 minutes - Cooking Time: 20 minutes - Servings: 8

Ingredients:

- 5 eggs, separated - 1/2 cup erythritol
- 1/4 cup unsweetened coconut milk
- 1/2 cup coconut flour
- 1/2 tsp baking powder
- 1/2 tsp vanilla
- 1/2 cup butter softened
- Pinch of salt

Directions:

1. Preheat the oven to 400 F. Grease cake pan and set aside.
2. In a bowl, beat sweetener and butter until smooth.
3. Add egg yolks, coconut milk, and vanilla and stir to combine.
4. Add baking powder, coconut flour, and salt and stir well.
5. In a separate bowl, beat egg whites until stiff peak forms.
6. Gently fold egg whites into the egg yolk mixture.
7. Pour batter in a prepared pan and bake for 20 minutes.
8. Slice and serve.

Nutrition: Calories 189 Fat 16.8 g Carbohydrates 5.8 g Sugar 0.5 g Protein 5 g Cholesterol 133 mg

39. EASY LEMON CHEESECAKE

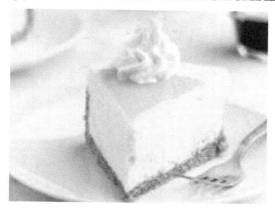

Preparation Time: 10 minutes - Cooking Time: 55 minutes - Servings: 8

Ingredients:

- 4 eggs - 2 tbsp. erythritol - 1/4 tsp lemon extract
- 1 fresh lemon juice - 18 oz. ricotta cheese - 1 fresh lemon zest

Directions:

1. Preheat the oven to 350 F. Grease cake pan and set aside.
2. In a large bowl, beat ricotta cheese until smooth. Add egg one by one and whisk well.
3. Add lemon juice, lemon extract, lemon zest, and sweetener and mix well.
4. Pour batter in the prepared cake pan and bake for 50-55 minutes.
5. Let it cool completely then place in the refrigerator for 2 hours.
6. Slice and serve.

Nutrition: Calories 120 Fat 7.3 g Carbohydrates 3.6 g Sugar 0.4 g Protein 10 g Cholesterol 102 mg

40. DELICIOUS POUND CAKE

Preparation Time: 10 minutes - Cooking Time: 35 minutes - Servings: 9

Ingredients:

- 5 eggs - 1 tsp orange extract - 1 cup Splenda - 4 oz. cream cheese, softened
- 1/2 cup butter, softened - 1 tsp baking powder - 6.5 oz. almond flour - 1 tsp vanilla

Directions:

1. Preheat the oven to 350 F. Grease 9-inch cake pan and set aside.
2. Add all ingredients into the mixing bowl and beat until fluffy.
3. Pour batter into the prepared pan and bake for 35-40 minutes.
4. Slice and serve.

Nutrition: Calories 295 Fat 27.3 g Carbohydrates 4.3 g Sugar 1 g Protein 4.1 g Cholesterol 132 mg

CANDY AND CONFECTIONS RECIPES

41. CHOCOLATE BONBONS

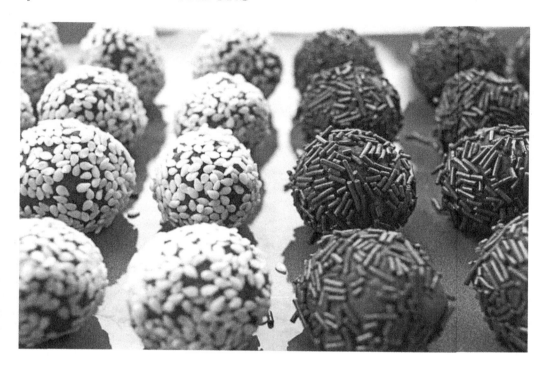

Preparation Time: 5 minutes - Cooking Time: 2 hours - Servings: 6

Ingredients:

- 5 tbsp. softened butter - 3 tbsp. coconut oil
- 2 tbsp. sugar-free raspberry syrup - 2 tbsp. cocoa powder

Directions:

1. Mix the entire batch of ingredients in a pan.
2. Empty the bombs into six molds or muffin tins.
3. Place the prepared tin into the freezer for a minimum of two hours. Enjoy!

Nutrition: Net Carbs 5.7 g Calories 164 Total Fat 14.7 g Saturated Fat 7.5 g Cholesterol 0 mg Sodium 2 mg Total Carbohydrate 7.7 g Fiber 2 g Total Sugars 4.6 g Protein 3.2 g Calcium 8 mg Iron 3 mg Potassium 145 mg

42. CHOCOLATE COCONUT BITES

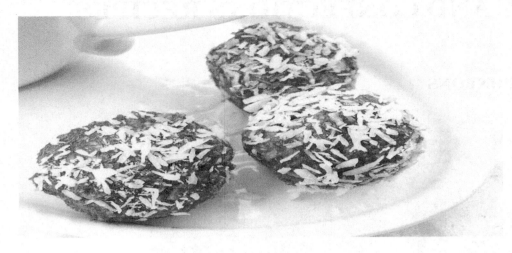

Preparation Time: 15 minutes - Cooking Time: 2 hours - Servings: 6

Ingredients:

- 4 oz. unsweetened 80% or higher dark chocolate
- 1/3 cup heavy cream
- 1 cup coconut flour
- 1 tbsp. chocolate protein powder
- ¼ cup shredded unsweetened coconut
- 4 tbsp. coconut oil

Directions:

1. Dice the dark chocolate into bits.
2. Warm up the heavy cream in a saucepan over medium-low.
3. Stir in the chocolate bits and coconut oil.
4. Continue stirring until combined and then remove from the burner.
5. Stir in the protein powder and coconut flour.
6. Store in the refrigerator for a minimum of two hours.
7. Take the dough out of the fridge when they are cool.
8. Shape into balls and roll through the shredded coconut until coated.
9. Store in the fridge in a closed container.

Nutrition: Net Carbs 8.2g Calories 237 Total Fat 18.5 Saturated Fat 12.8g Cholesterol 9mg Sodium 10mg Total Carbohydrate 19.7g Fiber 11.5g Total Sugars 0.4g Protein 5.5g Calcium 25m Iron 4mg Potassium 176mg

43. CHOCOLATE COVERED ALMONDS

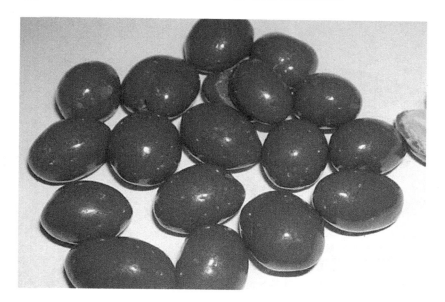

Preparation Time: 10 minutes - Cooking Time: 30 minutes - Servings: 5

Ingredients:

- 3/4 cup unsweetened dark chocolate baking chips
- 1½ cups whole raw almonds
- 1 tsp. pure vanilla extract
- 1 pinch sea salt

Directions:

1. Cut a piece of parchment paper to cover a baking tray.
2. Toss the chips into a saucepan using low heat. Stir and add the vanilla.
3. Once the chocolate is melted, add the almonds and stir until coated.
4. Arrange them on the baking tray and dust with the salt.
5. Place in the fridge for a minimum of 30 minutes before you are ready to devour.
6. For a change of taste, sprinkle with some ground cinnamon.

Nutrition: Net Carbs 4.6 g Calories 279 Total Fat 26.3 g Saturated Fat 8.7 g
Cholesterol 0 mg Sodium 49 mg Total Carbohydrate 11.8 g Fiber 7.2 g Total Sugars 1.3 g
Protein 9.2 g Calcium 85 mg Iron 3 mg Potassium 210 mg

44. ALMOND JOY

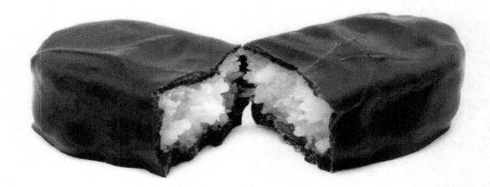

Preparation Time: 15 minutes - Cooking Time: 15 minutes - Servings: 6

Ingredients:

- 2 tsp. erythritol
- 8 oz. shredded coconut
- 4 oz. sugar-free dark chocolate chips
- ½ cup almonds (or any nut of your choice), raw or dry roasted

Directions:

1. Combine the shredded coconut with the sweetener in a medium-sized bowl; mix well until the coconut clumps together, for a couple of minutes.
2. Make small candies from the mixture, and place an almond in the middle of each one.
3. Now, melt the chocolate in the microwave or a double boiler.
4. Dip each candy into the chocolate and arrange it onto wax paper.
5. Put the coated candies into the freezer and let chill until set.
6. Serve and enjoy.

Nutrition: Net Carbs 14.8g Calories 260 Total Fat 23.1g Saturated Fat 15.5 Cholesterol 5mg Sodium 15mg Total Carbohydrate 21g Fiber 6.2g Total Sugars 4.3g Protein 3.5g Calcium 22mg Iron 6mg. Potassium 193mg

45. CANDY DOTS

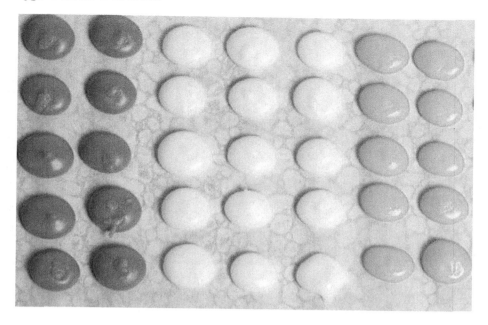

Preparation Time: 15 minutes - Cooking Time: 2 hours - Servings: 4

Ingredients:

- 1½ cups Allulose
- ¼ cup pasteurized egg white
- food coloring

Directions:

1. Using a hand mixer, whisk the egg white for a minute or two, until entirely frothy.
2. Slowly add in the Allulose; continue to whisk until peaks form.
3. Evenly divide the prepared mixture into bowls—as many as you want to color.
4. Slowly add the drops of color to each bowl until you achieve your desired color.
5. Mix until the color is uniform, and then transfer each color to a zippered sandwich bag.
6. Print template and place under each paper you will be piping onto.
7. Clip a tiny tip off one corner of each bag, and pipe dots onto unprinted sheets.
8. Let set for a couple of hours, and then cut the strips apart.

Nutrition: Net Carbs 8.5 g Calories 195 Total Fat 3.5 g Saturated Fat 1.5 g Cholesterol 0 mg Sodium 418 mg Total Carbohydrate 9 g Fiber 0.5 g Total Sugars 0 g Protein 26 g

46. PEANUT CANDY

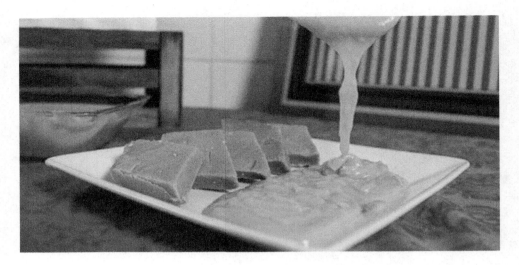

Preparation Time: 15 minutes - Cooking Time: 30 minutes - Servings: 10

Ingredients:

- ½ cup Allulose - 10 oz. peanut butter
- 1/3 cup low-carb corn syrup - butter & Swerve as required to coat pan
- 1 cup water - Sugar-free chocolate/candy coating

Directions:

1. Lightly grease a 10" or 12" skillet with some butter.
2. Mound the peanut butter in the middle of your skillet.
3. Coat a large-sized cookie sheet with Swerve (enough to cover).
4. Combine corn syrup with Allulose and water in a large pot or saucepan.
5. Cook until it reaches the hard crack on a candy thermometer.
6. Pour the mixture on top of the peanut butter; give everything a good stir.
7. Pour the mixture immediately over the prepared cookie sheet.
8. Immediately roll out to ½" to ¼" thickness.
9. Using a pizza cutter, cut it into desired rectangles.
10. Let completely cool.
11. You may coat with the tempered chocolate or melted candy coating.

Nutrition: Net Carbs 11.7g Calories 206 Total Fat 15.4g Saturated Fat 3.7g Cholesterol 3mg Sodium 139mg Total Carbohydrate 13.4g Fiber 1.7g Total Sugars 5.4g Protein 7.1g Calcium 2mg Iron 3mg Potassium 185 mg

47. BOSTON BAKED BEANS CANDY

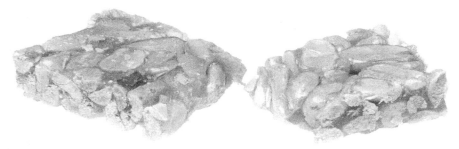

Preparation Time: 15 minutes - Cooking Time: 20 minutes - Servings: 6

Ingredients:

- 2 cups of raw peanuts - 1 cup Allulose - ½ cup water

Directions:

1. Place all the ingredients in a large skillet.
2. Cook over medium heat until the water is evaporated, stirring now and then.
3. Pour the mixture onto a large-sized cookie sheet, and bake in preheated 325°F oven for 20 minutes. Break apart, if required.

Nutrition: Net Carbs 3.8 g Calories 276 Total Fat 24 g Saturated Fat 3.3 g Cholesterol 0 mg Sodium 9 mg Total Carbohydrate 7.9 g Fiber 4.1 g Total Sugars 1.9 g Protein 12.6 g Calcium 45 mg Iron 2 mg Potassium 343 mg

48. TOOTSIE ROLL CANDY

Preparation time: 15 minutes - Cooking time: Refrigerate - Servings: 36

Ingredients:

- 1/4 cup cocoa - 1/4 cup whey protein, unflavored - 2 tbsp. whole milk powder
- 1/2 cup erythritol - 1/8 tsp. salt - 3 tbsp. Sukrin fiber syrup - 2 tbsp. butter, melted
- 1/2 tsp. vanilla extract

Directions:

1. Combine whey protein, cocoa, powdered milk, erythritol, and salt in a bowl and mix.
2. Set aside. Heat Sukrin fiber syrup in a microwave oven for 30 seconds.
3. Add the vanilla extract and melted butter. Add in the cocoa mix and combine well until crumbly. Flatten the dough and cut into strips.
4. Roll the strips into a rope about the diameter of the tootsie roll. Cut the rope strips into tootsie roll sizes.
5. Wrap each roll individually on a small wax paper. Refrigerate until ready to serve.

Nutrition: Calories: 120 Carbs: 28 g Fat: 3 g Protein: 1 g

49. CARAMEL CHEWY CANDY

Preparation time: 5 minutes - Cooking time: 10 minutes - Servings: 12

Ingredients:

- 2 tbsp. choc zero syrup
- 2 tsp. monk fruit sweetener, powder
- 1 tbsp. butter, unsalted

Directions:

1. On low heat, melt the butter.
2. After melting the butter, turn to medium-low heat add the syrup and the monk fruit.
3. Bring to a boil. Whisk often past the boiling point.
4. Once the mixture starts to froth, turn off the heat and continue to whisk for another 20 seconds.
5. Pour in silicone molds and let it cool.
6. Serve as is or wrapped in wax paper.

Nutrition: Calories: 170 Carbs: 28 g Fat: 6 g Protein: 1 g

50. HARD NOUGAT CANDY

Preparation time: 10 minutes - Cooking time: 2 hours and 50 minutes - Servings: 12

Ingredients:

- 1 cup macadamia nuts - 1 cup erythritol - 2 tbsp. water - 1 egg white, large - A pinch of salt

Directions:

1. Preheat oven to 200 degrees F. Prepare an 8x6-inch pan and line with parchment paper.
2. In a skillet over medium heat, toast the macadamia nuts until golden. Remove from heat.
3. In a small saucepan, combine water and erythritol. Stir on a medium heat until translucent and simmering, about 20 minutes.
4. While waiting to simmer, beat the egg white and salt until it starts to form soft peaks.
5. Pour the syrup in slowly while you continually whisk the egg whites until they are well combined.
6. Move back to the sauce pan then keep stirring over low heat for about 30 minutes. Pour over the macadamia nuts.
7. Place the bake pan in the oven for 2 hours to dry the candy.
8. Remove from the oven and allow cooling at room temperature before unmolding and slicing into pieces.

Nutrition: Calories: 40 Carbs: 10 g Fat: 5 g Protein: 0 g

51. CHEWY SALTWATER TAFFY

Preparation time: 15 minutes - Cooking time: 30 minutes - Servings: 100

Ingredients:

- 1/2 cup water - 1 cup light corn syrup - 2 cups sweetener, granulated - 3/4 tsp. salt
- 2 tbsp. butter - 1 tsp. vanilla extract - 1/4 cup marshmallow cream – 3 drops food coloring

Directions:

1. At medium-high heat, combine water, corn syrup, sweetener, and salt. Stir until sugar dissolves. With a pastry brush, wash down the side of the saucepan to prevent crystallization.
2. Bring to a boil without stirring until it reaches 255 degrees F to get a soft chewy taffy. Increase temperature by 5 to 10 degrees to get a firm to very firm taffy.
3. Remove from heat once you reach the desired temperature, add the butter, vanilla and stir until butter completely melts. Spread out the mixture in a baking sheet.
4. Pour the marshmallow cream and the food color on top. Let the candy cool for 5 to 10 minutes. Fold all edges to the center of the marshmallow cream.
5. Knead the candy until marshmallow cream and food color mix in. Stretch the candy into a rope then bring it back together. Twist the candy and repeat the pulling process.
6. Continue to pull and twist for 20 minutes until it holds its shape well or until you see parallel ridges on the candy.
7. Divide the taffy into manageable working sizes. Roll them into long thin ropes of 1/2-inch diameter then cut them into 1-inch size piece.
8. Wrap in wax paper to keep it from sticking together and serve.

Nutrition: Calories: 15 Total Fat: 0 Total Carbohydrates: 3 g Net Carbohydrates: 3 g Protein: 0

52. CLASSIC GUMMY BEARS

Preparation time: 15 minutes - Cooking time: 30 minutes - Servings: 2

Ingredients:

- 0.3 oz. packet Jell-O, sugar free - 0.25 oz. packet unflavored gelatin powder - 1/4 cup water

Directions:

1. Prepare gummy bear molds that have 50 molds per tray.
2. Combine all ingredients in a cooking pan. Cook over low heat until powder completely dissolves. Remove from stove the use a dropper to fill up the mold.
3. Once all empty molds are filled, place in the refrigerator around 30 minutes until the gelatin sets. Pop the bears off the tray and serve.
4. You can use different flavor packs of Jell-O and add the same amount of unflavored gelatin and water, then repeat the process.

Nutrition: Calories: 110 Carbs: 24 g Fat: 0 g Protein: 2 g

53. RASPBERRY SOUR GUMMY BEARS

Preparation time: 15 minutes - Cooking time: 45 minutes - Servings: 6

Ingredients:

- 1/2 cup water - 2 tbsp. raspberry powder – 2/4 tbsp. allulose
- 1/2 tsp. vitamin c powder - 2 1/2 tbsp. unflavored gelatin

For the sour coating:

- 2 tsp. allulose - 1/2 tsp. raspberry powder - 1/4 tsp. vitamin c powder

Directions:

1. Over medium heat, use a saucepan to combine water, raspberry powder, allulose, and vitamin c and stir.
2. Turn to low and add in gelatin. Stir for 3 minutes until powder dissolves.
3. Remove from heat and pour into a bowl.
4. Use a dropper to fill in the gummy bear silicone mold.
5. Allow to cool for 15 minutes before placing in the refrigerator for 30 minutes.
6. Mix all the sour coating ingredients.
7. Coat gummies before serving.

Nutrition: Calories: 100 Carbs: 24 g Fat: 0 g Protein: 1 g

54. COKE FLAVORED GUMMY

Preparation time: 15 minutes - Cooking time: 1 – 2 hours - Servings: 5

Ingredients:

- 25 g gelatin powder, unflavored - 1/3 cup boiling water
- 1/2 cup cold water - 12 drops stevia cola flavor
- 9 drops natural purple food coloring - 3 drops natural yellow food coloring

Directions:

1. In a microwaveable container, place boiling water and add gelatin powder.
2. Whisk then place in microwave for 30 seconds. Remove from microwave and whisk again.
3. Add the cold water and continue whisking to combine. Add the cola drops and whisk.
4. Taste if you wish to add more flavoring. Add both the food colors to get a dark brown color.
5. Place in coke bottle molds and remove bubbles on the poured mixture.
6. Chill for 1 to 2 hours before popping them out of the mold.

Nutrition: Calories: 14 Calories from Fat: 0 Total Fat: 0 g Total Carbohydrates: 0 g

Net Carbohydrates: 0 g Protein: 3.5 g

55. FRUITY ORANGE JELLY CANDY

Preparation time: 15 minutes - Cooking time: 3 hours - Servings: 81

Ingredients:

- 2 tsp. butter - 3/4 oz. powdered fruit pectin - 1/2 tsp. baking soda
- 3/4 cup water - 1 cup sweetener, granulated - 1 cup light corn syrup
- 1/8 tsp. orange oil - 5 drops red food color - 5 drops yellow food color

Directions:

1. Line a 9x9-inch pan with two tsp. of butter.
2. Combine the pectin, baking soda, and water in a large saucepan.
3. The mixture will look foamy. Bring to a boil.
4. In a separate saucepan, combine sweetener and corn syrup.
5. Bring the mixture to a boil, around 4 minutes.
6. Slowly add in in the boiled pectin mixture on the sweetener mixture and boil for one minute while stirring constantly.
7. Remove from heat. Stir in the orange oil and food coloring.
8. Pour onto the 9-inch pan immediately and let it stand for 3 hours under room temperature.
9. Dip a knife in warm water and slice the firm jelly into 1-inch square sizes.
10. Place on a rack and let it stand uncovered at room temperature overnight.

Nutrition: Calories: 130 Carbs: 39 g Fat: 0 g Protein: 0 g

56. CREAMY ORANGE GUMMY

Preparation time: 10 minutes - Cooking time: 1 – 2 hours - Servings: 4

Ingredients:

- 0.3 oz. Jell-O orange, sugar-free - 2 envelopes unflavored gelatin
- 1 tbsp. swerve powdered sweetener - 1/2 cup cold water - 1/2 cup heavy cream

Directions:

1. Soften the unflavored gelatin in cold water. Simmer the cream on medium heat.
2. Add Jell-O and sweetener and mix until dissolved.
3. Pour the softened gelatin and mix until dissolved.
4. Remove from heat and pour in candy silicone mold or pour in a loaf pan and cut after it sets. Chill 1-2 hours before removing from mold. Keep refrigerated before serving.

Nutrition: Calories: 119 Calories from Fat: 99 Total Fat: 11 g Total Carbohydrates: 1 g

Net Carbohydrates: 1 g Protein: 2 g

57. CUCUMBER LIME GUMMY

Preparation time: 10 minutes - Cooking time: 2 hours - Servings: 4

Ingredients:

- 225 g cucumber - 3g mint tea leaves - 1/2 lime juice - 10 g gelatin powder - A dash of stevia

Directions:

1. Combine all the ingredients except gelatin then put in a blender. Strain the mixture into a small pot. Turn on stove at medium heat and start to simmer the mixture.
2. Add in the gelatin powder slowly and stir until completely dissolved. Strain the gelatin mixture into a clean container. Chill for 2 hours. Pop out from tray to serve.

Nutrition: Calories: 80 Carbs: 21 g Fat: 0 g Protein: 0 g

58. VANILLA GUMDROPS

Preparation time: 10 minutes - Cooking time: 2 hours - Servings: 7

Ingredients:

- 5 cups filtered water - 2 tbsp. dried vanilla leaves - 1/4 tsp. citric acid - 1 pinch ginger
- 1 tbsp. grated lemon zest - 6 micro-scoops stevia extract - 6 tbsp. beef gelatin, grass fed
- 1/2 cup water - 2 tsp. vanilla extract - 4 drops yellow food coloring

Directions:

1. Infuse the vanilla leaves in 5 cups of water by boiling it for 5 minutes. Cool before straining and transferring to another pan. Place the strained vanilla water back on the stove to heat again. Combine 1/2 cup water and gelatin and add to the vanilla water. Stir and let it boil until the gelatin dissolves. Remove from heat. Add the sweetener, citric acid, lemon zest, and ginger. Mix until it turns into a golden hue. Divide the mixture into 2 and add vanilla flavor and yellow food color on the one half. Freeze mixture for 2 hours in a silicon mold. Remove the gumdrops from your mold before serving.

Nutrition: Calories: 130 Carbs: 33 g Fat: 0 g Protein: 0 g

59. BLACKBERRY CANDY

Preparation time: 5 minutes - Cooking time: Refrigerate - Servings: 8

Ingredients:

- 1/4 cup cashew butter - 1 tbsp. fresh lemon juice - 1/2 cup fresh blackberries
- 1/2 cup coconut oil - 1/2 cup unsweetened coconut milk

Directions:

1. Heat cashew butter, coconut oil, and coconut milk in a skillet over medium-low heat until warm. Transfer the cashew nut mixture to the blender along with the remaining ingredients and mix until smooth. Pour the mixture into the silicone candy mold and refrigerate until set. Serve and enjoy.

Nutrition: Calories: 203 kcal Fat: 21.2 g Protein: 1.9 g Carbohydrates: 3.9 g Fiber: 1 g

60. SWEET GREEN COCONUT

Preparation Time: 15 minutes - Cooking Time: 0 minutes - Servings: 24
Ingredients:

- Vanilla Extract (1 t.) - Spinach (2 C.) - Avocados (2) - Coconut Milk (1 C.)

Directions:

1. If you need to get more fats and more nutrients into your diet for the day, these fat bombs will be perfect for you. It should be noted that while these aren't as sweet as some of the other fat bombs you will see, they are still excellent to incorporate into your diet!

2. To make these fat bombs, all you will need to do is place all of the ingredients from the list above into a blender and blend on a high speed until everything becomes smooth.

3. Once you have your mixture, you will want to spoon it into your silicone molds or lined muffin tins. When this is in place, pop it into the freezer for two hours, and they will be ready after that.

Nutrition: Calories: 50 Fats: 5 g Proteins: 2 g Carbs: 1 g

61. COCONUT MACADAMIA CANDY

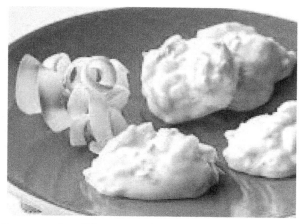

Preparation Time: 5 minutes - Cooking Time: 2 hours - Servings: 14

Ingredients:

- 1/2 cup coconut oil - 1/2 tsp. vanilla extract - 1 cup macadamia nuts
- 2 tbsp. swerve - 8 drops liquid stevia

Directions:

1. Add every ingredient into a blender and blitz until smooth.

2. Pour mixture into the silicone candy mold and place in the refrigerator for 2 hours or until candy is hardened. Serve and enjoy.

Nutrition: Calories: 137 kcal Fat: 15 g Protein: 0.8 g Carbohydrates: 1.6 g Fiber: 0.8 g

COOKIES RECIPES

62. CHOCOLATE CHIP COOKIES

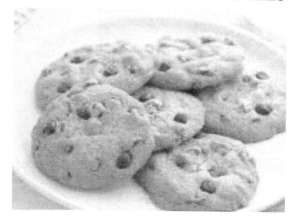

Preparation Time: 10 minutes - Cooking Time: 15 minutes - Servings: 24

Ingredients:

- 1 large egg - 2/3 cup sweetener (such as Swerve) - 5½ tbsp. butter (room temperature)
- ½ tsp. vanilla extract - 1¼ cups almond flour - 1/8 tsp. sea salt (optional)
- 1½ tsp. baking powder - 1 tbsp. coconut flour - ¼ cup chopped pecans (optional)
- ½ cup sugar-free chocolate chips

Directions:

1. Use some parchment paper or silicone baking mats to line two baking sheets. Set the oven temperature to 325°F.
2. Use a mixer to blend the sweetener and butter. Then mix in the egg and vanilla extract until well combined.
3. In another bowl, combine the two flours, sea salt, and baking powder, stirring until blended.
4. Combine the contents of the two bowls; stir well.
5. Fold in the pecans and chocolate chips. Arrange the cookie dough by the tablespoonful into the prepared pans. They should be approximately 1½ inches apart.
6. Bake until the bottoms are browned or about 12-15 minutes. Let them cool until firm and set (approximately 30 minutes).

Nutrition: Net Carbs 9.8 g Calories 69 Total Fat 5.1 g Saturated Fat 1.1 g Cholesterol 8 mg

Sodium 19mg Total Carbohydrate 10.9 g Fiber 1.1 g Total Sugars 8.7 g Protein 2.1 g Calcium 23 mg

63. CHOCOLATE COCONUT COOKIES

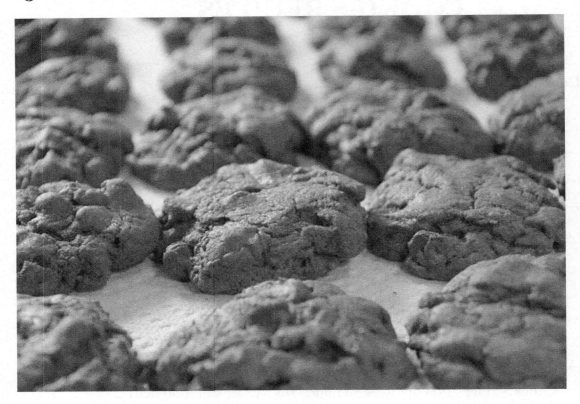

Preparation Time: 10 minutes - Cooking Time: 20 minutes - Servings: 20

Ingredients:

- 1 cup almond flour - 3 tbsp. coconut flour - ¼ tsp. salt
- 1/3 cup unsweetened shredded coconut - 1/3 cup Erythritol - ½ tsp. baking powder
- ¼ cup cocoa powder - ¼ cup coconut oil - ¼ tsp. vanilla extract - 2 eggs

Directions:

1. Preheat oven to 350°F. Cover a baking tin with some parchment paper.
2. Combine the dry ingredients and mix with a hand mixer.
3. In another bowl, combine the wet components, and then add to the dry until well blended.
4. Break apart pieces of the cookie dough and roll into 20 balls.
5. Arrange on the cookie sheet and bake for 15-20 minutes until done.

Nutrition: Net Carbs 4.4 g Calories 54 Total Fat 4.7 g Saturated Fat 3.2 g Cholesterol 16 mg Sodium 38 mg Total Carbohydrate 5.9 g Fiber 1.5 g Total Sugars 0.2 g Protein 1.4 g Calcium 12 mg Iron 1 mg Potassium 51 mg

64. COCONUT NO-BAKE COOKIES

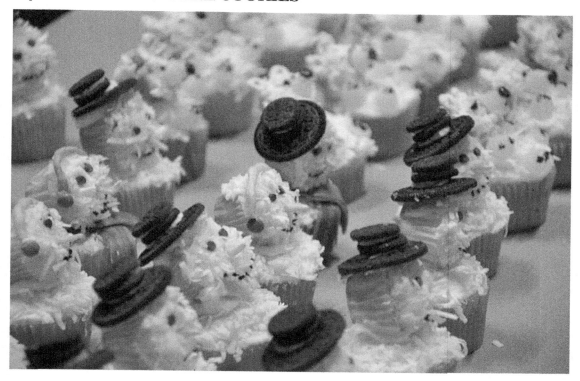

Preparation Time: 10 minutes - Servings: 20

Ingredients:

- 1 cup melted coconut oil
- 1 packet (2g) Monk fruit sweetener
- 3 cups shredded unsweetened coconut flakes

Directions:

1. Cut out a sheet of parchment paper and place it on a cookie tray.
2. Combine all of the fixings. Run your hands through some water from the tap, and then shape the mixture into small balls. Arrange them on the pan around 1"-2" apart.
3. Press them down to form a cookie, and refrigerate until firm.
4. You can prepare these into individual bags if you're an on-the-go kind of person. They will stay fresh covered for up to 7 days (room temperature). Store in the fridge for up to a month, or frozen up to two months.

Nutrition: Net Carbs 1.3 g Calories 106 Total Fat 10.8 g Saturated Fat 5.8 g Cholesterol 0 mg Sodium 68 mg Total Carbohydrate 2.5 g Fiber 1.2 g Total Sugars 0 g Protein 0.6 g Calcium 6 mg Iron 0 mg Potassium 0 mg

65. CREAM CHEESE COOKIES

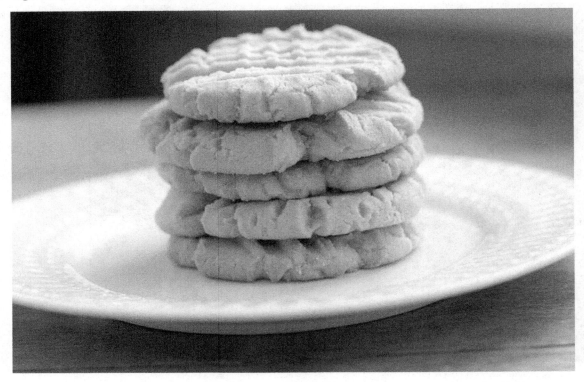

Preparation time: 10 minutes - Cooking Time: 4 hours - Servings: 4

Ingredients:

- 3/4 cup low-carb sugar-free maple syrup - 4 oz. softened cream cheese
- 1 cup butter - 1 egg - ½ cup coconut flour - 2 cups almond flour

Directions:

1. Preheat oven to 350°F.
2. Cream the sweetener and butter until fluffy. Fold in the cream cheese and add the egg.
3. Stir in both flours and mix in the vanilla.
4. Chill the prepared dough for a minimum of four hours.
5. Squeeze the dough into a cookie press. You can also roll it into a log and slice.
6. For pressed cookies, bake 8-10 minutes; for sliced cookies, 10-12 minutes.

Nutrition: Net Carbs 11 g Calories 1286 Total Fat 128.1 g Saturated Fat 78.6 g Cholesterol 164 mg Sodium 364 mg Total Carbohydrate 22.9 g Fiber 12 g Total Sugars 0.2 g Protein 17.9 g Calcium 39 mg Iron 1 mg Potassium 59 mg

66. GINGER SNAP COOKIES

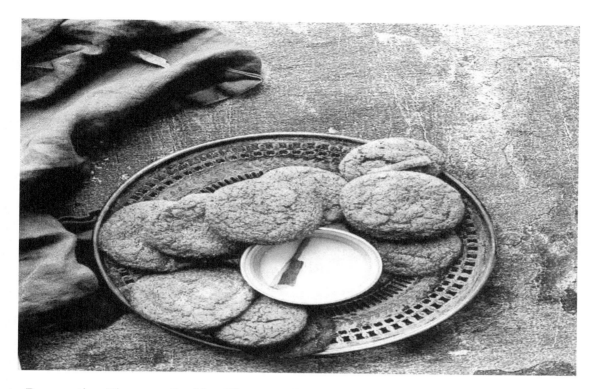

Preparation Time: 5 - Cooking Time: 11 minutes - Servings: 3

Ingredients:

- ¼ tsp. ground cloves - ¼ tsp. nutmeg - ¼ tsp. salt - 2 cups almond flour
- ½ tsp. ground cinnamon - ¼ cup unsalted butter - 1 tsp. vanilla extract - 1 large egg

Directions:

1. Preheat the oven to 350°F.
2. Whisk the dry components in a mixing bowl.
3. Blend in the rest of the ingredients into the dry mixture using a hand blender.
4. The dough will be stiff.
5. Measure out the dough for each cookie and flatten with a fork or your fingers.
6. Bake for about 9-11 minutes or until browned.

Nutrition: Net Carbs 2.5 g Calories 270 Total Fat 26.3 g Saturated Fat 10.9 g Cholesterol 95 mg Sodium 331 mg Total Carbohydrate 4.8 g Fiber 2.3 g Total Sugars 1 g Protein 6.1 g Calcium 58 mg Iron 1 mg Potassium 31 mg

67. NUT BUTTER COOKIES

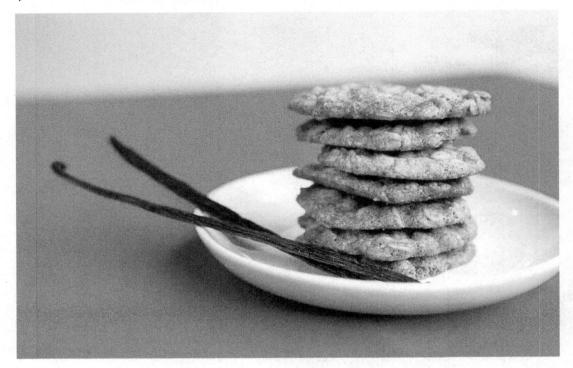

Preparation Time: 10 minutes - Cooking Time: 12 minutes - Servings: 10

Ingredients:

- 8½ oz. almond butter - ¼ cup Erythritol
- 1 egg - 2½ cups almond flour
- ¼ tsp. salted butter - ¼ cup raw coconut butter

Directions:

1. Preheat the oven to 320°F. Prepare a cookie sheet with a sheet of parchment paper.
2. Using a double boiler, melt the almond butter.
3. Take it from the heat and stir in the flour, coconut butter, Erythritol, salt, and egg.
4. Fold until well mixed.
5. Break into 10 segments and roll into balls.
6. Place on the prepared pan and flatten with a fork or your hand.
7. Bake for 12 minutes until browned to your liking.

Nutrition: Net Carbs 10.6 g Calories 296 Total Fat 25.1 g Saturated Fat 5 g Cholesterol 17 mg Sodium 20 mg Total Carbohydrate 16 g Fiber 5.4 g Total Sugars 7 g Protein 9.8 g

68. ORANGE WALNUT COOKIES

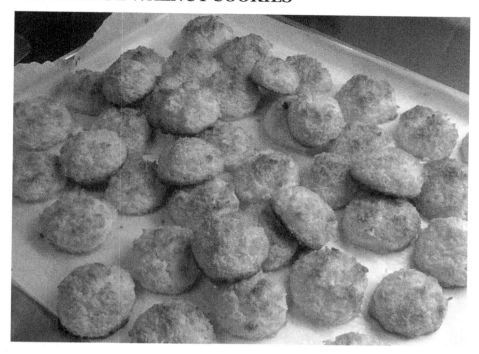

Preparation Time: 10 minutes - Cooking Time: 50 minutes - Servings: 10

Ingredients:

- 8 oz. walnut halves - 3 tbsp. zested minced orange - 1 egg
- 20 Stevia drops - 4 tbsp. cinnamon (for garnish)
- 2 tbsp. shredded coconut (for garnish)

Directions:

1. Preheat oven to 320°F. Toast the walnuts for about 10 minutes until browned.
2. Add them to a food processor.
3. Toss in the rest of the fixings and continue blending until it is smooth.
4. Shape into 10 balls and slightly flatten.
5. Sprinkle with some shredded coconut. Bake for 40 minutes.
6. Cool on the rack a few minutes and add to a platter to finish cooling.
7. Store in an air-tight container and enjoy it.

Nutrition: Net Carbs 1 g Calories 152 Total Fat 14 g Saturated Fat 1 g Cholesterol 16 mg Sodium 7 mg Total Carbohydrate 3.4 g Fiber 2.4 g Total Sugars 0.3 g Protein 6.1 g Calcium 28 mg Iron 1 mg Potassium 128 mg

69. NO BAKE CHOCO PEANUT BUTTER COOKIES

Preparation Time: 10 minutes - Cooking Time: 10 minutes - Servings: 12

Ingredients:

- 2/3 cup creamy peanut butter - 1/2 cup almonds, chopped - 1/2 tsp vanilla
- 3 tbsp. unsweetened cocoa powder - 1/2 cup erythritol

Directions:

1. Line baking sheet with parchment paper and set aside.
2. Add cocoa powder and sweetener into the food processor and process until mix.
3. Add vanilla and peanut butter and process until smooth.
4. Add almonds and process until just combined.
5. Scoop cookies onto a prepared baking sheet and gently press down.
6. Place in refrigerator for 1 hour or until hardened.
7. Serve and enjoy.

Nutrition: Calories 111 Fat 9.4 g Carbohydrates 4.4 g Sugar 1.6 g Protein 4.7 g Cholesterol 0 mg

70. CREAM CHEESE PUMPKIN COOKIES

Preparation Time: 10 minutes - Cooking Time: 25 minutes - Servings: 16

Ingredients:

- 1/2 cup pumpkin puree - 1 1/2 tsp pumpkin spice - 1 tsp vanilla - 1/2 cup erythritol
- 1/2 cup butter, softened - 3 oz. cream cheese - 1/2 cup coconut flour - Pinch of salt

Directions:

1. Preheat the oven to 350 F.
2. Line baking sheet with parchment paper and set aside.
3. In a mixing bowl, whisk together butter and sweetener.
4. Add pumpkin puree, vanilla, and cream cheese and whisk until smooth.
5. Add the pumpkin spice, coconut flour, and salt and mix until well combined.
6. Make small balls from the mixture and arrange on a prepared baking sheet.
7. Gently press down the balls using a spoon.
8. Bake cookies for 25 minutes. Once done then let it cool completely.
9. Serve and enjoy.

Nutrition: Calories 88 Fat 8.2 g Carbohydrates 2.9 g Sugar 0.6 g Protein 1.1 g Cholesterol 21 mg

71. EASY BUTTER COOKIES

Preparation Time: 10 minutes - Cooking Time: 10 minutes - Servings: 10

Ingredients:

- 3 tbsp. butter, softened
- 1/4 cup erythritol
- 1 cup almond flour
- 1/2 tsp vanilla

Directions:

1. Preheat the oven to 350 F.
2. Line baking sheet with parchment paper and set aside.
3. Add all ingredients into the mixing bowl and mix until well combined.
4. Make 1-inch balls from mixture and place on a prepared baking sheet.
5. Using a fork flatten each ball and bake for 10 minutes.
6. Once cookies have done then remove from oven and let them cool completely.
7. Serve and enjoy.

Nutrition: Calories 98 Fat 8.8 g Carbohydrates 2.4 g Sugar 0 g Protein 2.4 g Cholesterol 9 mg

72. LEMON CREAM CHEESE COOKIES

Preparation Time: 10 minutes - Cooking Time: 10 minutes - Servings: 18

Ingredients:

- 1 egg - 2 tbsp. fresh lemon juice - 6 oz. cream cheese - 1/3 cup erythritol
- 1/2 cup coconut flour - 3 tbsp. coconut oil, melted - 1 tsp vanilla

Directions:

1. Preheat the oven to 350 F.
2. Line baking sheet with parchment paper and set aside.
3. In a medium bowl, add egg, lemon juice, cream cheese, coconut oil, and vanilla and mix using a hand mixer until well combined.
4. Add coconut flour and sweetener and mix everything well.
5. Make small balls from mixture and place on a prepared baking sheet and using a fork lightly flatten the cookies.
6. Bake cookies for 10 minutes.
7. Let the cookies cool completely then serve.

Nutrition: Calories 71 Fat 6.2 g Carbohydrates 2.7 g Sugar 0.1 g Protein 1.5 g Cholesterol 19 mg

73. CINNAMON ALMOND COOKIES

Preparation Time: 10 minutes - Cooking Time: 15 minutes - Servings: 24

Ingredients:

- 1 egg - 1 cup almond flour - 1 tsp cinnamon - 1/2 cup coconut flour - 1 tsp vanilla
- 1/4 cup erythritol - 1/2 cup butter - 1/4 tsp nutmeg - 1/2 cup ground pecans - 1/2 tsp salt

Directions:

1. Add ground pecans and almond flour in a pan and cook over medium heat for 3-5 minutes or until fragrant.
2. Remove pan from heat. Add nutmeg, cinnamon, and salt and stir well and let it cool.
3. In a large bowl, beat butter and sweetener until smooth. Stir in vanilla and egg.
4. Add coconut flour and almond flour mixture and mix until dough is formed.
5. Cover dough and place in the refrigerator for 1 hour.
6. Preheat the oven to 350 F. Line baking sheet with parchment paper and set aside.
7. Remove cookie dough from the refrigerator. Make 24 small balls from dough and place on a prepared baking sheet.
8. Lightly flatten balls with the fork and bake for 12-15 minutes.
9. Let the cookies cool completely then serve.

Nutrition: Calories 97 Fat 8.7 g Carbohydrates 3.2 g Sugar 0.2 g Protein 1.9 g Cholesterol 17 mg

74. EASY PEANUT BUTTER COOKIES

Preparation Time: 10 minutes - Cooking Time: 12 minutes - Servings: 8

Ingredients:

- 1 egg
- 1 cup creamy peanut butter
- 1/2 cup Swerve

Directions:

1. Preheat the oven to 350 F.
2. Line baking sheet with parchment paper and set aside.
3. Add all ingredients into the bowl and mix until well combined.
4. Make small balls from mixture and place on a prepared baking sheet.
5. Gently flatten the balls using a fork.
6. Bake cookies for 10-12 minutes.
7. Let the cookies cool completely then serve.

Nutrition: Calories 198 Fat 16.8 g Carbohydrates 6.5 g Sugar 3.1 g Protein 8.8 g Cholesterol 20 mg

75. NUTRITIOUS COCONUT COOKIES

Preparation Time: 10 minutes Cooking Time: 15 minutes Servings: 18

Ingredients:

- 1 1/2 cups shredded coconut flakes - 2 tbsp. water - 2 tbsp. coconut oil
- 1 tsp cinnamon - 1 tsp vanilla - 10 drops liquid stevia
- 1/2 cup protein powder - 1/2 cup sunflower seeds, roughly chopped

Directions:

1. Preheat the oven to 300 F.
2. Line baking sheet with parchment paper and set aside.
3. Add all ingredients into the mixing bowl and mix until well combined.
4. If the mixture is too crumbly then add 1 tablespoon of oil.
5. Scoop cookies onto a prepared baking sheet and gently flatten using a fork.
6. Bake cookies for 15 minutes.
7. Let the cookies cool completely then serve.

Nutrition: Calories 55 Fat 4.6 g Carbohydrates 1.7 g Sugar 0.6 g Protein 2.4 g Cholesterol 6 mg

76. SIMPLE ALMOND FLOUR COOKIES

Preparation Time: 10 minutes Cooking Time: 12 minutes Servings: 12

Ingredients:

- 1 cup almond flour
- 1 tbsp. water
- 2 tbsp. coconut oil, melted
- 2 1/2 tbsp. Swerve
- Pinch of salt

Directions:

1. Preheat the oven to 350 F.
2. Line baking sheet with parchment paper and set aside.
3. Add all ingredients into the mixing bowl and mix until well combined.
4. Make 1-inch balls from mixture and place on a prepared baking sheet.
5. Gently flatten each ball using a fork.
6. Bake cookies for 10-12 minutes.
7. Let the cookies cool completely then serve.

Nutrition: Calories 77 Fat 6.7 g Carbohydrates 2.4 g Sugar 0 g Protein 2 g Cholesterol 0 mg

77. NO BAKE CHOCO COCONUT COOKIES

Preparation Time: 10 minutes - Cooking Time: 10 minutes - Servings: 12

Ingredients:

- 1 1/3 cup unsweetened shredded coconut - 1 tsp vanilla
- 1/4 cup unsweetened cocoa powder - 1/4 cup heavy whipping cream
- 1/4 cup creamy peanut butter - 1/2 cup Swerve

Directions:

1. Line baking sheet with parchment paper and set aside.
2. Add cocoa powder, heavy cream, peanut butter, sweetener, and vanilla in a non-stick saucepan and heat over medium-low heat for 2 minutes. Stir constantly.
3. Turn off the heat. Add shredded coconut and stir until well combined.
4. Make small balls from mixture and place on a prepared baking sheet and gently flatten with the spatula.
5. Refrigerate for 2 hours or until cookie hardened.
6. Serve and enjoy.

Nutrition: Calories 121 Fat 11 g Carbohydrates 5 g Sugar 1.4 g Protein 2.5 g Cholesterol 3 mg

78. FUDGY BROWNIE COOKIES

Preparation Time: 10 minutes - Cooking Time: 12 minutes - Servings: 14

Ingredients:

- 1 egg - 1/4 cup unsweetened chocolate chips - 1/2 cup erythritol
- 1/4 cup unsweetened cocoa powder - 1 cup almond butter, smooth

Directions:

1. Preheat the oven to 350 F.
2. Line baking sheet with parchment paper and set aside.
3. In a mixing bowl, mix the almond butter, egg, sweetener, and cocoa powder until well combined. If your batter is crumbly then add 2-3 tablespoon of almond milk.
4. Make sure batter looks fudgy, not runny and soft.
5. Add chocolate chips and stir well.
6. Make small balls from mixture and place on a prepared baking sheet.
7. Lightly press down each ball.
8. Bake cookies for 10-12 minutes.
9. Let the cookies cool completely then serve.

Nutrition: Calories 44 Fat 3.5 g Carbohydrates 2.2 g Sugar 0.1 g Protein 1.5 g Cholesterol 12 mg

79. CHOCO CHIP COCONUT COOKIES

Preparation Time: 10 minutes - Cooking Time: 17 minutes - Servings: 20

Ingredients:

- 2 eggs, lightly beaten - 1/3 cup coconut oil, melted
- 1/4 cup unsweetened chocolate chips - 1/4 cup erythritol
- 2 1/2 cups unsweetened shredded coconut - Pinch of salt

Directions:

1. Preheat the oven to 350 F.
2. Line baking sheet with parchment paper and set aside.
3. In a mixing bowl, mix shredded coconut, sweetener, and salt.
4. Add coconut oil, vanilla, chocolate chips, and eggs and stir until dough is formed.
5. Scoop cookies onto a prepared baking sheet and gently flatten using a fork.
6. Bake cookies for 17 minutes.
7. Let the cookies cool completely then serve.

Nutrition: Calories 142 Fat 13.7 g Carbohydrates 4 g Sugar 0.9 g Protein 1.8 g Cholesterol 16 mg

80. EASY PECAN SHORTBREAD COOKIES

Preparation Time: 10 minutes - Cooking Time: 10 minutes - Servings: 20

Ingredients:

- 1/2 cup pecans, chopped - 1 tsp vanilla - 1/2 tsp xanthan gum
- 3/4 cup Swerve - 1 stick butter, softened - 1 1/4 cups almond flour

Directions:

1. Preheat the oven to 350 F.
2. Line baking sheet with parchment paper and set aside.
3. In a mixing bowl, beat butter, sweetener, vanilla, xanthan gum, and almond flour until smooth.
4. Add pecans and stir well.
5. Make 1-inch balls from mixture and place on a prepared baking sheet.
6. Gently flatten each ball using a fork.
7. Bake cookies for 8-10 minutes.
8. Let the cookies cool completely then serve.

Nutrition: Calories 109 Fat 10.6 g Carbohydrates 2.2 g Sugar 0.2 g Protein 2 g Cholesterol 12 mg

81. NO BAKE ALMOND COOKIES

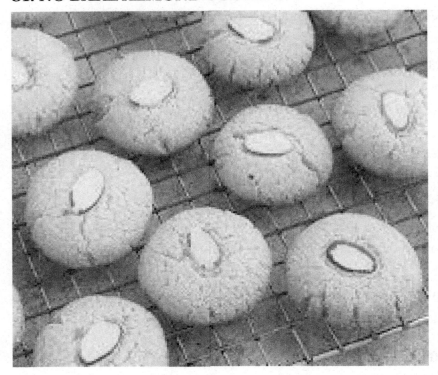

Preparation Time: 10 minutes - Cooking Time: 10 minutes - Servings: 12

Ingredients:

- 1.75 oz. Butter - 1/2 cup stevia - 1/2 cup peanut butter
- 1/2 cup shredded coconut - 1 cup flaked almonds

Directions:

1. Line baking sheet with parchment paper and set aside.
2. In a mixing bowl, mix flaked almonds and shredded coconut.
3. In a small pan, add butter, stevia, and peanut butter and heat over medium heat until butter is melted.
4. Pour melted butter mixture over the almond mixture and stir well to combine.
5. Drop a tablespoon of mixture per cookie onto the prepared baking sheet.
6. Place in refrigerator for 2 hours or until cookies harden.
7. Serve and enjoy.

Nutrition: Calories 161 Fat 14.7 g Carbohydrates 3.6 g Sugar 1.7 g Protein 4.8 g Cholesterol 9 mg

BUNS AND MUFFINS RECIPES

82. CINNAMON ROLL MUFFINS

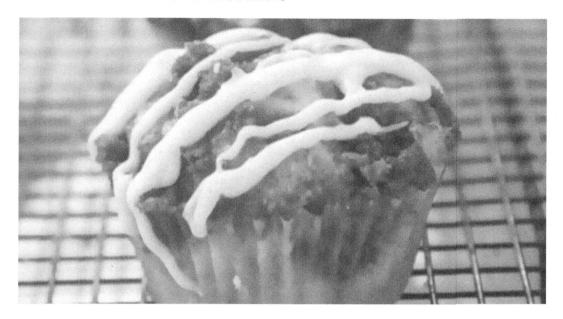

Preparation Time: 5 minutes - Cooking Time: 15 minutes - Servings: 6

Ingredients:

- ½ cup almond flour - 2 scoops vanilla protein powder - 1 tsp baking powder
- 1 tbsp. cinnamon - ½ cup almond butter - ½ cup pumpkin puree - ½ cup coconut oil

For the Glaze

- ¼ cup coconut butter - ¼ cup milk of choice
- 1 tbsp. granulated sweetener - 2 tsp lemon juice

Directions:

1. Let your oven preheat at 350 degrees F. Layer a 12-cup muffin tray with muffin liners.
2. Add all the dry ingredients to a suitable mixing bowl then whisk in all the wet ingredients.
3. Mix until well combined then divide the batter into the muffin cups.
4. Bake them for 15 minutes then allow the muffins to cool on a wire rack.
5. Prepare the cinnamon glaze in a small bowl then drizzle this glaze over the muffins.

Nutrition: Calories 252 Total Fat 17.3 g Saturated Fat 11.5 g Cholesterol 141 mg Sodium 153 mg Total Carbs 7.2 g Sugar 0.3 g Fiber 1.4 g Protein 5.2 g

83. MUFFINS WITH BLUEBERRIES

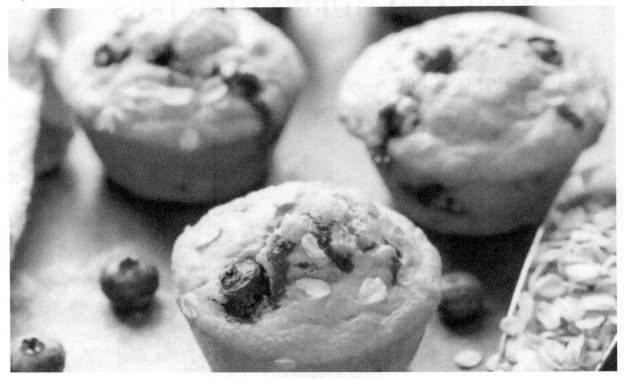

Preparation Time: 10 minutes - Cooking Time: 25 minutes - Servings: 8

Ingredients:

- 3/4 cup coconut flour - 6 eggs - ½ cup coconut oil, melted
- 1/3 cup unsweetened coconut milk - ½ cup fresh blueberries
- 1/3 cup granulated sweetener - 1 tsp vanilla extract - 1 tsp baking powder

Directions:

1. Preheat your oven at 356 degrees F.
2. Mix coconut flour with all the other ingredients except blueberries in a mixing bowl until smooth.
3. Stir in blueberries and mix gently.
4. Divide this batter in a greased muffin tray evenly.
5. Bake the muffins for 25 minutes until golden brown.

Nutrition: Calories 195 Total Fat 14.3 g Saturated Fat 10.5 g Cholesterol 175 mg

Sodium 125 mg Total Carbs 4.5 g Sugar 0.5 g Fiber 0.3 g Protein 3.2 g

84. CHOCOLATE ZUCCHINI MUFFINS

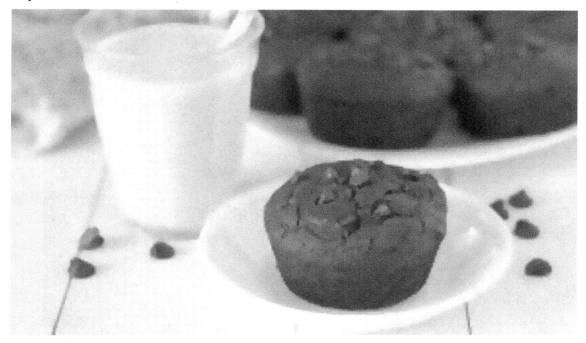

Preparation Time: 10 minutes - Cooking Time: 30 minutes - Servings: 9

Ingredients:

- ½ cup coconut flour - 3/4 tsp baking soda - 2 tbsp. cocoa powder - ½ tsp salt
- 1 tsp cinnamon - ½ tsp nutmeg - 3 large eggs - 2/3 cup Swerve sweetener
- 2 tsp vanilla extract - 1 tbsp. oil - 1 medium zucchini, grated - ¼ cup heavy cream
- 1/3 cup Lily's chocolate baking chips

Directions:

1. Preheat your oven at 356 degrees F.
2. Layer a 9-cup o muffin tray with muffin liners then spray them with cooking oil.
3. Whisk coconut flour with salt, cinnamon, nutmeg, sweetener, baking soda, and cocoa powder in a bowl.
4. Beat eggs in a separate bowl then add oil, cream, vanilla, and zucchini.
5. Stir in the coconut flour mixture and mix well until fully incorporated.
6. Fold in chocolate chips then divide the batter into the lined muffin cups.
7. Bake these muffins for 30 minutes then allow them to cool on a wire rack.

Nutrition: Calories 151 Total Fat 14.7 g Saturated Fat 1.5 g Cholesterol 13 mg Sodium 53 mg Total Carbs 1.5 g Sugar 0.3 g Fiber 0.1 g Protein 0.8 g

85. BLACKBERRY-FILLED LEMON MUFFINS

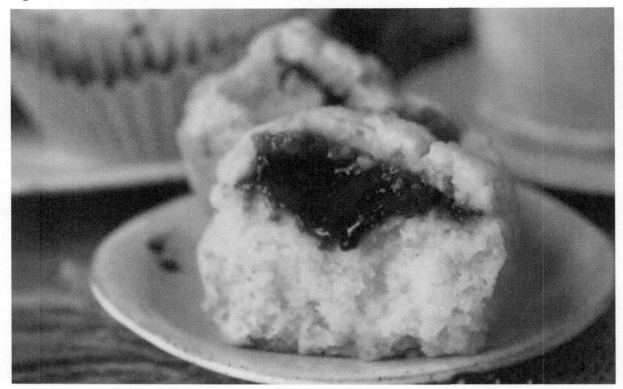

Preparation Time: 5 minutes - Cooking Time: 30 minutes - Servings: 12

Ingredients:

For the Blackberry Filling:

- 3 tbsp. granulated stevia
- 1 tsp lemon juice
- ¼ tsp xanthan gum
- 2 tbsp. water
- 1 cup fresh blackberries

For the Muffin Batter:

- 2 ½ cups super fine almond flour
- 3/4 cup granulasted stevia
- 1 tsp fresh lemon zest
- ½ tsp sea salt
- 1 tsp grain-free baking powder
- 4 large eggs

- ¼ cup unsweetened almond milk
- ¼ cup butter
- 1 tsp vanilla extract
- ½ tsp lemon extract

Directions:

For the Blackberry Filling:

1. Add granulated sweetener and xanthan gum in a saucepan.
2. Stir in lemon juice and water then place it over the medium heat.
3. Add blackberries and stir cook on low heat for 10 minutes.
4. Remove the saucepan from the heat and allow the mixture to cool.

For the Muffin Batter:

5. Preheat your oven at 356 degrees F and layer a muffin tray with paper cups.
6. Mix almond flour with salt, baking powder, lemon zest, baking powder, and sweetener in a mixing bowl.
7. Whisk in eggs, vanilla extract, lemon extract, butter, and almond milk.
8. Beat well until smooth. Divide half of this batter into the muffin tray.
9. Make a depression at the center of each muffin.
10. Add a spoonful of blackberry jam mixture to each depression.
11. Cover the filling with remaining batter on top.
12. Bake the muffins for 30 minutes then allow them to cool.
13. Refrigerate for a few hours before serving.
14. Enjoy.

Nutrition: Calories 261 Total Fat 7.1 g Saturated Fat 13.4 g Cholesterol 0.3 mg Sodium 10 mg Total Carbs 6.1 g Sugar 2.1 g Fiber 3.9 g Protein 1.8 g

86. BANANA MUFFINS

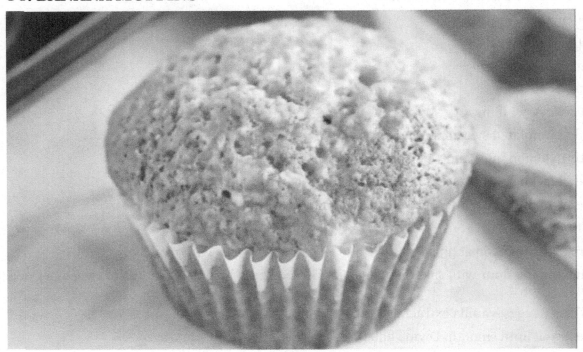

Preparation Time: 10 minutes - Cooking Time: 18 minutes - Servings: 12

Ingredients:

- 3 large eggs - 2 cups bananas, mashed (3-4 medium bananas)
- ½ cup almond butter (peanut butter can also be used)
- ¼ cup butter (olive oil can also be used) - 1 tsp vanilla
- ½ cup coconut flour (almond flour can also be used)
- 1 tbsp. cinnamon - 1 tsp baking powder - 1 tsp baking soda
- Pinch sea salt - ½ cup chocolate chips

Directions:

1. Preheat your oven at 356 degrees F. Line a 12-cup muffin tray with paper liners.
2. Whisk eggs with almond butter, vanilla, butter, and mashed bananas in a large bowl.
3. Stir in coconut flour, baking soda, cinnamon, baking powder, and salt. Mix well with a wooden spoon.
4. Divide this batter into the muffin cups then bake them for 18 minutes.
5. Allow them to cool then refrigerate for 30 minutes. Enjoy.

Nutrition: Calories 139 Total Fat 4.6 g Saturated Fat 0.5 g Cholesterol 1.2 mg Sodium 83 mg Total Carbs 7.5 g Sugar 6.3 g Fiber 0.6 g Protein 3.8 g

87. BREAKFAST BUNS

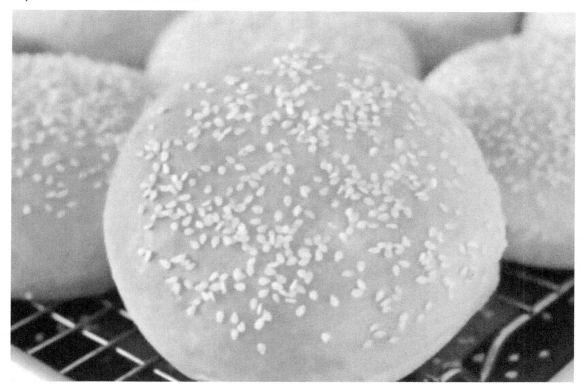

Preparation Time: 10 minutes - Cooking Time: 25 minutes - Servings: 4

Ingredients:

- 3 egg whites, room temperature - 1 egg, room temperature
- ¼ cup boiling hot water - ¼ cup almond flour - ¼ cup coconut flour
- 1 tbsp. psyllium husk powder - 1 tsp baking powder - Sesame seeds, for sprinkling

Directions:

1. Preheat your oven at 356 degrees F.
2. Add everything to a food processor and blend for 20 seconds until smooth.
3. Let it sit for 20 minutes then divide the dough into 4 equal parts.
4. Shape the dough into buns then place them on a baking sheet lined with wax paper.
5. Score the top of each bun with a fork and sprinkle sesame seeds on top.
6. Bake the buns for 25 minutes until golden brown.
7. Enjoy.

Nutrition: Calories 200 Total Fat 11.1 g Saturated Fat 9.5 g Cholesterol 124.2 mg Sodium 46 mg Total Carbs 1.1 g Sugar 1.3 g Fiber 0.4 g Protein 0.4 g

88. DINNER ROLLS

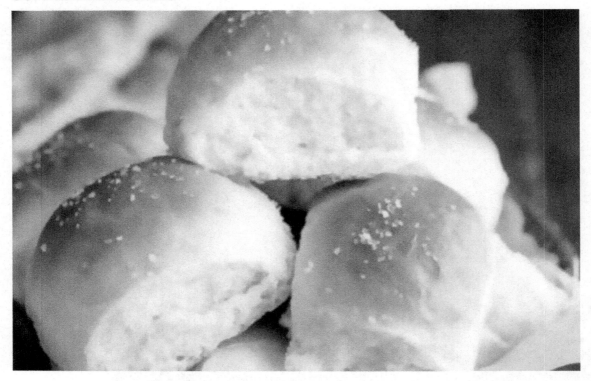

Preparation Time: 5 minutes - Cooking Time: 12 minutes - Servings: 8

Ingredients:

- 1 cup mozzarella, shredded - 1 oz. cream cheese - 1 cup almond flour
- ¼ cup ground flaxseed - 1 egg - ½ tsp baking soda

Directions:

1. Preheat your oven at 400 degrees F. Layer a baking sheet with wax paper and set it aside.
2. Melt mozzarella and cream cheese in a medium bowl by heating the mixture for 1 minute in the microwave.
3. Mix well then add the egg. Whisk well until combined.
4. Add baking soda, flaxseed, and almond flour.
5. Mix well to form a smooth dough then make 6 balls out of this dough.
6. Place the balls on the baking sheet lined with wax paper.
7. Sprinkle sesame seeds over the balls.
8. Bake them for 12 minutes until golden brown. Enjoy.

Nutrition: Calories 136 Total Fat 10.7 g Saturated Fat 0.5 g Cholesterol 4 mg Sodium 45 mg Total Carbs 1.2 g Sugar 1.4 g Fiber 0.2 g Protein 0.9

89. BUNS WITH PSYLLIUM HUSK

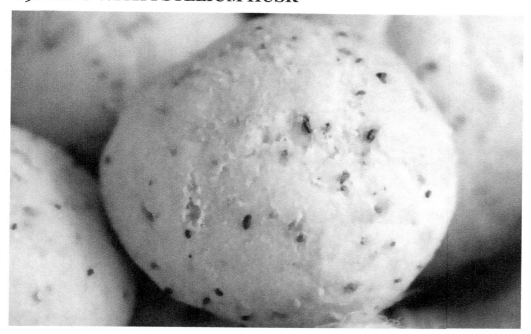

Preparation Time: 15 minutes - Cooking Time: 30 minutes - Servings: 5

Ingredients:

- 4 tbsp. boiling water

Dry Ingredients

- oz. blanched almond flour - 2 tbsp. psyllium husk powder - 1 tsp baking powder
- 1 tsp black sesame seeds - 1 tsp white sesame seeds - 2 tsp sunflower seeds
- 1 tsp black chia seeds - ½ tsp Himalayan salt - ½ tsp garlic powder

Wet Ingredients

- 1 egg - 2 egg whites - 1 tbsp. apple cider vinegar - 3 tbsp. melted refined coconut oil

Directions:

1. Preheat your oven at 356 degrees F.
2. Add dry ingredients to a bowl along with wet ingredients. Mix well until smooth.
3. Slowly add boiled water into the dough and mix well to absorb the water.
4. Divide the dough into 5 balls, grease them with cooking oil. And roll them in your hands.
5. Place the balls on a baking sheet lined with parchment paper.
6. Bake them for 30 minutes until golden. Enjoy.

Nutrition: Calories 76 Total Fat 7.2 g Saturated Fat 6.4 g Cholesterol 134 mg Sodium 8 mg
Total Carbs 2g Sugar 1 g Fiber 0.7 g Protein 2.2 g

90. FATHEAD ROLLS

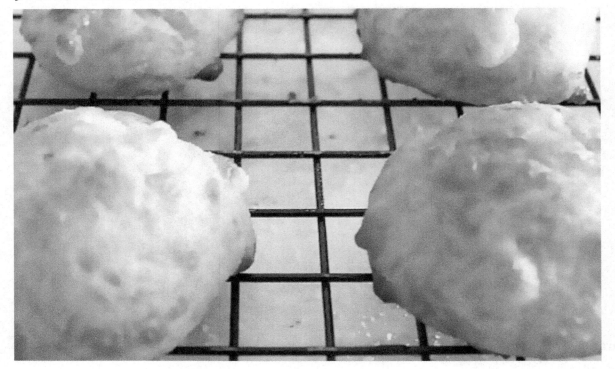

Preparation Time: 5 minutes - Cooking Time: 12 minutes - Servings: 6

Ingredients:

- 2 oz. cream cheese - 3/4 cup shredded mozzarella - 1 egg beaten - ¼ tsp garlic powder
- 1/3 cup almond flour - 2 tsp baking powder - ½ cup shredded cheddar cheese

Directions:

1. Preheat your oven at 425 degrees F.
2. Heat mozzarella and cream cheese in a small bowl for 20 seconds in the microwave.
3. Beat egg with all the dry ingredients in a separate bowl.
4. Stir in cheese mixture to make a sticky dough adding the cheddar cheese at the end.
5. Mix well then wrap the dough in plastic wrap.
6. Refrigerate this dough for 30 minutes then divide it into 4 equal parts.
7. Cut each ball in half and place them flat side down on a baking sheet lined with wax paper.
8. Bake them for 12 minutes until golden.
9. Enjoy.

Nutrition: Calories 193 Total Fat 10 g Saturated Fat 13.2 g Cholesterol 120 mg Sodium 8 mg
Total Carbs 2.5 g Sugar 1 g Fiber 0.7 g Protein 2.2 g

91. CINNAMON STRAWBERRY MUFFINS

Preparation Time: 10 minutes - Cooking Time: 20 minutes - Servings: 12

Ingredients:

- 3 eggs - 1/3 cup heavy cream - 1 tsp vanilla - 1/2 cup Swerve
- 2/3 cup strawberries, diced - 1 tsp cinnamon - 2 tsp baking powder
- 2 1/2 cups almond flour - 5 tbsp. butter, melted - Pinch of salt

Directions:

1. Preheat the oven to 350 F. Line muffin tin with cupcake liners.
2. In a bowl, beat together butter and swerve.
3. Add eggs, cream, and vanilla and beat until frothy.
4. Sift together almond flour, cinnamon, baking powder, and salt.
5. Add almond flour mixture to the wet ingredients and mix until well combined.
6. Add strawberries and stir well.
7. Pour mixture into the muffin cups and bake for 20 minutes.
8. Serve and enjoy.

Nutrition: Calories 208 Fat 18 g Carbohydrates 6 g Sugar 1.3 g Protein 6.6g Cholesterol 58 mg

92. PECAN MUFFINS

Preparation Time: 10 minutes - Cooking Time: 20 minutes - Servings: 12

Ingredients:

- 4 eggs - 1 tsp vanilla - 1/4 cup almond milk - 2 tbsp. butter, melted
- 1/2 cup swerve sweetener - 1 tsp psyllium husk - 1 tbsp. baking powder
- 1 1/2 cups almond flour - 1/2 cup pecans, chopped - 1/2 tsp ground cinnamon
- 2 tsp allspice

Directions:

1. Preheat the oven to 400 F. Line muffin tin with cupcake liners.
2. Beat eggs, almond milk, vanilla, sweetener, and butter in a bowl until smooth.
3. Add remaining ingredients and mix until well combined.
4. Pour mixture into the muffin cups and bake for 15-20 minutes.
5. Serve and enjoy.

Nutrition: Calories 205 Fat 18 g Carbohydrates 6 g Sugar 1 g Protein 6 g Cholesterol 60 mg

93. COCONUT ZUCCHINI MUFFINS

Preparation Time: 10 minutes - Cooking Time: 25 minutes - Servings: 8

Ingredients:

- 6 eggs - 4 drops liquid stevia - 1/4 cup Swerve
- 1/3 cup coconut oil, melted
- 1 cup zucchini, grated
- 3/4 cup coconut flour
- 1/4 tsp ground nutmeg
- 1 tsp ground cinnamon
- 1/2 tsp baking soda

Directions:

1. Preheat the oven to 350 F. Line muffin tin with cupcake liners.
2. Add all ingredients except zucchini in a bowl and mix well.
3. Add zucchini and stir well.
4. Pour mixture into the muffin cups and bake for 25 minutes.
5. Serve and enjoy.

Nutrition: Calories 135 Fat 12.6 g Carbohydrates 2 g Sugar 0.6 g Protein 4.5 g Cholesterol 123 mg

94. MOIST RASPBERRY MUFFINS

Preparation Time: 10 minutes - Cooking Time: 20 minutes - Servings: 12

Ingredients:

- 3 large eggs - 1/3 cup coconut oil, melted - 1 1/2 tsp gluten-free baking powder
- 1/2 cup erythritol - 2 1/2 cups almond flour - 3/4 cup raspberries
- 1/2 tsp vanilla - 1/3 cup unsweetened almond milk

Directions:

1. Preheat the oven to 350 F. Line muffin tin with cupcake liners.
2. In a large bowl, stir together almond flour, baking powder, erythritol.
3. Mix in the coconut oil, vanilla, eggs, and almond milk. Fold in raspberries.
4. Pour mixture into the muffin cups and bake for 20 minutes.
5. Serve and enjoy.

Nutrition: Calories 217 Fat 19 g Carbohydrates 6 g Sugar 2 g Protein 7 g Cholesterol 47 mg

95. MOIST & FLUFFY PUMPKIN MUFFINS

Preparation Time: 10 minutes - Cooking Time: 25 minutes - Servings: 10

Ingredients:

- 4 large eggs - 1 tbsp. gluten-free baking powder
- 2/3 cup erythritol - 1/2 cup almond flour
- 1 tsp vanilla - 1/3 cup coconut oil, melted
- 1/2 cup pumpkin puree - 1 tbsp. pumpkin pie spice
- 1/2 cup coconut flour - 1/2 tsp sea salt

Directions:

1. Preheat the oven to 350 F. Line muffin tin with cupcake liners.
2. In a large bowl, stir together coconut flour, pumpkin pie spice, baking powder, erythritol, almond flour, and sea salt.
3. Stir in eggs, vanilla, coconut oil, and pumpkin puree until well combined.
4. Pour mixture into the muffin cups and bake for 25 minutes.
5. Serve and enjoy.

Nutrition: Calories 151 Fat 13 g Carbohydrates 7 g Sugar 2 g Protein 5 g Cholesterol 74 mg

96. DELICIOUS CAPPUCCINO MUFFINS

Preparation Time: 10 minutes - Cooking Time: 25 minutes - Servings: 12

Ingredients:

- 4 eggs - 1/2 cup Swerve - 2 cups almond flour
- 1/2 tsp vanilla - 1 tsp espresso powder
- 1 tsp cinnamon - 2 tsp baking powder
- 1/4 cup coconut flour - 1/2 cup sour cream - 1/4 tsp salt

Directions:

1. Preheat the oven to 350 F. Line muffin tin with cupcake liners.
2. Add sour cream, vanilla, espresso powder, and eggs in a blender and blend until smooth.
3. Add almond flour, cinnamon, baking powder, coconut flour, sweetener, and salt and blend to combine.
4. Pour mixture into the muffin cups and bake for 25 minutes.
5. Serve and enjoy.

Nutrition: Calories 151 Fat 13 g Carbohydrates 5 g Sugar 0.8 g Protein 6.2 g Cholesterol 59 mg

97. LEMON BLUEBERRY MUFFINS

Preparation Time: 10 minutes - Cooking Time: 25 minutes - Servings: 12

Ingredients:

- 2 large eggs - 1 tsp baking powder
- 5 drops stevia - 1/4 cup butter, melted
- 1 cup heavy cream - 2 cups almond flour
- 1/4 tsp lemon zest - 1/2 tsp lemon extract
- 1/2 cup fresh blueberries

Directions:

1. Preheat the oven to 350 F. Line muffin tin with cupcake liners.
2. Add eggs to the mixing bowl and whisk until well mix.
3. Add remaining ingredients to the eggs and mix well to combine.
4. Pour mixture into the muffin cups and bake for 25 minutes.
5. Serve and enjoy.

Nutrition: Calories 191 Fat 17 g Carbohydrates 5 g Sugar 1 g Protein 5.4 g Cholesterol 55 mg

98. FLAXSEED PUMPKIN MUFFINS

Preparation Time: 10 minutes - Cooking Time: 2 minutes - Servings: 2

Ingredients:

- 1 egg - 2 tbsp. swerve - 2 tbsp. ground flaxseed
- 2 tbsp. almond flour - 1 1/2 tsp pumpkin spice
- 1/4 tsp baking powder - 2 tbsp. pumpkin puree

Directions:

1. In a bowl, mix together pumpkin puree and egg.
2. In another bowl, mix together almond flour, pumpkin spice, baking powder, sweetener, and ground flaxseed.
3. Pour pumpkin and egg mixture into the almond flour mixture and mix well.
4. Pour mixture into the 2 ramekins and microwave for 1-2 minutes.
5. Serve and enjoy.

Nutrition: Calories 132 Fat 9 g Carbohydrates 8 g Sugar 1 g Protein 6 g Cholesterol 82 mg

99. INSTANT POT MOIST CARROT MUFFINS

Preparation Time: 10 minutes - Cooking Time: 20 minutes - Servings: 8

Ingredients:

- 3 eggs - 1/4 cup coconut oil, melted - 1 cup almond flour
- 1/2 cup pecans, chopped - 1/2 cup heavy cream - 1 tsp apple pie spice
- 1 cup shredded carrot - 1/3 cup Swerve - 1 tsp baking powder

Directions:

1. Pour 1 1/2 cups of water into the instant pot then place a trivet in the pot.
2. Add all ingredients except pecans and carrots into the mixing bowl and blend until fluffy.
3. Add carrots and pecans and fold well.
4. Pour batter into the silicone muffin molds and place it on top of the trivet.
5. Seal pot with lid and cook on high pressure for 20 minutes.
6. Once done then release pressure using the quick-release method. Remove lid.
7. Serve and enjoy.

Nutrition: Calories 300 Fat 29.3 g Carbohydrates 7.2 g Sugar 1.8 g Protein 6.9 g Cholesterol 72 mg

100. INSTANT POT BROWNIE MUFFINS

Preparation Time: 10 minutes - Cooking Time: 15 minutes - Servings: 4

Ingredients:

- 4 eggs - 1/2 cup unsweetened cocoa powder - 1 cup almond flour - 1/2 cup coconut oil
- 1 tsp vanilla - 1/4 cup unsweetened dark chocolate, chopped - 1/4 cup Swerve

Directions:

1. Pour 1 cup of water into the instant pot then place a trivet in the pot.
2. In a mixing bowl, beat together eggs, coconut oil, vanilla, and swerve until creamy.
3. Add cocoa powder, chocolate, and almond flour to the egg mixture and mix well.
4. Pour batter into the ramekins and cover ramekins with foil.
5. Place ramekins on top of the trivet.
6. Seal pot with lid and cook on high pressure for 15 minutes.
7. Once done then allow to release pressure naturally. Remove lid.
8. Serve and enjoy.

Nutrition: Calories 466 Fat 44 g Carbohydrates 11 g Sugar 0.9 g Protein 11 g Cholesterol 164 mg

101. INSTANT POT CHOCOLATE MUFFINS

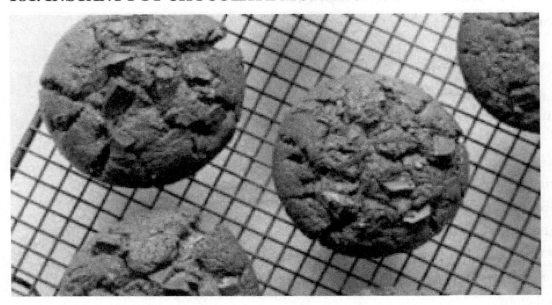

Preparation Time: 10 minutes - Cooking Time: 10 minutes - Servings: 6

Ingredients:

2 eggs - 3 tbsp. yogurt - 1/4 cup cream cheese - 1 cup shredded coconut

1 1/2 cups almond flour - 1 tsp vanilla - 1/4 cup blueberries - 2 tsp baking powder

3 tbsp. butter - 2 tbsp. unsweetened cocoa powder - 1/4 cup Swerve

Directions:

1. In a large bowl, add butter and eggs and beat until fluffy.
2. Add swerve, yogurt, and cream cheese and stir well.
3. Add almond flour, baking powder, and shredded coconut. Mix well.
4. Add blueberries and fold well.
5. Pour batter into the silicone muffin molds and set aside.
6. Pour 1 cup of water into the instant pot and place trivet in the pot.
7. Place silicone molds on top of the trivet.
8. Seal pot with lid and cook on high pressure for 10 minutes.
9. Once done then release pressure using quick release. Remove lid.
10. Serve and enjoy.

Nutrition: Calories 330 Fat 29 g Carbohydrates 11 g Sugar 3.2 g Protein 10 g Cholesterol 81 mg

CUSTARD & MOUSSE RECIPES

102. RASPBERRY MOUSSE

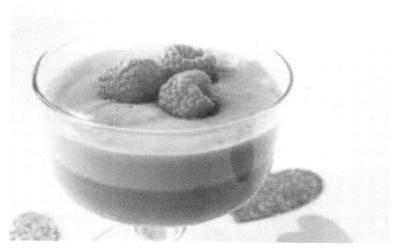

Preparation time: 10 minutes - Cooking time: 20 minutes - Servings: 4

Ingredients:

- 2 cups coconut cream
- 1 cup raspberries
- Juice of 1 lime
- 1 teaspoon vanilla extract
- 1 tablespoon stevia

Directions:

1. Combine all ingredients, pulse well in the blender, divide into cups and serve cold.

Nutrition: Calories: 298 Fat: 28.8 g Fiber: 4.7 g Carbs: 11.4 g Protein: 3.2 g

103. VANILLA BLUEBERRIES MOUSSE

Preparation time: 10 minutes - Cooking time: 20 minutes - Servings: 4

Ingredients:

- 1 cup heavy cream - ½ cup almond milk - 1 cup blueberries
- 3/4 teaspoon vanilla stevia - ½ teaspoon vanilla extract

Directions:

1. In a blender, combine cream with the berries, milk and the other ingredients, pulse well, divide into bowls and serve.

Nutrition: Calories 195 Fat 18.4 g Fiber 1.5 g Carbs 7.8 g Protein 1.6 g

104. LIME MOUSSE

Preparation time: 10 minutes - Cooking time: 20 minutes - Servings: 4

Ingredients:

- Zest of 1 lime, grated - Juice of 1 lime - 1 cup heavy cream
- 1 cup coconut cream - 1 teaspoon almond extract - 1 tablespoon stevia

Directions:

1. In a blender, lime juice with lime zest and the other ingredients, pulse well, divide into small cups and serve.

Nutrition: Calories: 249 Fat: 25.4 g Fiber: 1.4 g Carbs: 5.2 g Protein: 2 g

105. COCOA MOUSSE

Preparation time: 10 minutes - Cooking time: 20 minutes - Servings: 4

Ingredients:

- 2 tablespoons cocoa powder
- 1 cup heavy cream
- ½ cup coconut milk
- 1 tablespoon stevia

Directions:

1. In a blender, mix the cream with the cocoa and the other ingredients, pulse well and divide into bowls.
2. Serve cold.

Nutrition: Calories: 178 Fat: 18.6 g Fiber: 1.5 g Carbs: 4 g Protein: 1.8 g

106. VANILLA COCOA MOUSSE

Preparation time: 10 minutes - Cooking time: 20 minutes - Servings: 2

Ingredients:

- 1 cup coconut milk
- 2 tablespoons cocoa powder
- 1 cup heavy cream
- 1 tablespoon stevia
- 1 teaspoon vanilla extract

Directions:

1. In a blender, combine the milk with the cocoa and the other ingredients, pulse well, divide into bowls and serve cold.

Nutrition: Calories: 501 Fat: 51.5 g Fiber: 4.3 g Carbs: 11.6 g Protein: 5 g

107. COCONUT MOUSSE

Preparation time: 10 minutes - Cooking time: 20 minutes - Servings: 4

Ingredients:

- 2 tablespoons coconut flakes, unsweetened
- 1 cup coconut cream
- ½ cup coconut milk
- 1 tablespoon stevia

Directions:

1. Combine all ingredients in a blender, pulse well, divide into bowls and serve.

Nutrition: Calories: 216 Fat: 22.3 g Fiber: 2.2 g Carbs: 5.9 g Protein: 2.2 g

108. CINNAMON MOUSSE

Preparation time: 10 minutes - Cooking time: 20 minutes - Servings: 4

Ingredients:

- 1 cup heavy cream - 1 tablespoon stevia - 2 teaspoons cinnamon powder
- 1 cup coconut milk - ½ cup coconut cream - 1 teaspoon vanilla extract

Directions:

1. In a blender, mix the cream with the cinnamon, stevia and the other ingredients, pulse well, divide into bowls and serve cold.

Nutrition: Calories: 314 Fat: 32.6 g Fiber: 2 g Carbs: 6 g Protein: 2.7 g

109. MIXED BERRIES MOUSSE

Preparation time: 10 minutes - Cooking time: 20 minutes - Servings: 2

Ingredients:

- 1 cup heavy cream - 1 cup strawberries - 1 cup raspberries
- 1 cup blackberries - ½ cup blueberries - 1 tablespoon stevia - ½ teaspoon vanilla extract

Directions:

1. Combine all ingredients in a blender, pulse well, divide into bowls and serve cold.

Nutrition: Calories: 301 Fat: 19.1 g Fiber: 0.3 g Carbs: 1.9 g Protein: 4 g

110. SWEET GHEE MOUSSE

Preparation time: 10 minutes - Cooking time: 2 0 minutes - Servings: 4

Ingredients:

- 1 teaspoon almond extract
- ½ teaspoon vanilla extract
- 3 tablespoons ghee, melted
- 1 cup coconut cream
- 1 cup almond milk
- ½ tablespoon swerve

Directions:

1. In a blender, combine the ghee with the cream, milk and the other ingredients, pulse well, divide into bowls and serve.

Nutrition: Calories: 453 Fat: 48.1 g Fiber: 2.9 g Carbs: 7.3 g Protein: 2.9 g

111. CREAM CHEESE MOUSSE

Preparation time: 10 minutes - Cooking time: 20 minutes - Servings: 4

Ingredients:

- 1 cup coconut cream
- 1 tablespoon stevia
- 1 teaspoon almond extract
- 1 tablespoon lime zest, grated
- 1 cup cream cheese

Directions:

1. Combine all ingredients, pulse it in the blender then divide into bowls and serve.

Nutrition: Calories: 332 Fat: 31.4 g Fiber: 0.5 g Carbs: 9.2 g Protein: 5 g

112. NUTMEG MOUSSE

Preparation time: 2 hours - Cooking time: 20 minutes - Servings: 2

Ingredients:

- 1 teaspoon nutmeg, ground
- ½ teaspoon almond extract
- 1 cup almond milk
- 2 cups heavy cream

Directions:

1. In a blender, combine the milk with the nutmeg and the other ingredients, whisk and keep freeze for 2 hours.

Nutrition: Calories: 243 Fat: 22 g Fiber: 0 g Carbs: 6.2 g Protein: 4 g

113. LIME WATERMELON MOUSSE

Preparation time: 10 minutes - Cooking time: 20 minutes - Servings: 2

Ingredients:

- 1 cup watermelon, peeled and cubed
- 1 teaspoon lime zest, grated
- 1 cup almond milk
- 1 tablespoon lime juice
- 2 tablespoons stevia

Directions:

1. Combine watermelon and milk, lime zest and the other ingredients, pulse well, divide into bowls and serve.

Nutrition: Calories: 178 Fat: 4.4 g Fiber: 2 g Carbs: 3 g Protein: 5 g

114. PLUMS AND STRAWBERRIES MOUSSE

Preparation time: 10 minutes - Cooking time: 20 minutes - Servings: 2

Ingredients:

- 2 tablespoons stevia - 1 cup strawberries, chopped
- 1 cup plums, pitted and halved - juice of 1 lime - 1 cup coconut cream

Directions:

1. In a blender, combine the plums with the strawberries and the other ingredients, pulse well, divide into bowls and serve.

Nutrition: Calories: 400 Fat: 23 g Fiber: 4 g Carbs: 6 g Protein: 7 g

115. CHOCOLATE MOUSSE

Preparation time: 20 minutes - Cooking time: 20 minutes - Servings: 2

Ingredients:

- ½ cup heavy cream - ½ cup dark chocolate, unsweetened and melted
- 1 cup coconut milk - 1 tablespoon stevia - ½ teaspoon cinnamon powder

Directions:

1. In a blender, combine all ingredients then divide into bowls and keep in the fridge for 20 minutes before serving.

Nutrition: Calories: 78 Fat: 1 g Fiber: 1 g Carbs: 2 g Protein: 0 g

116. VANILLA CREAM CHEESE MOUSSE

Preparation time: 10 minutes - Cooking time: 20 minutes - Servings: 2

Ingredients:

- 1 teaspoon vanilla extract - 1 cup coconut cream - 2 ounces cream cheese
- 1 tablespoon ghee, melted - 1 tablespoon stevia

Directions:

1. In your blender, mix the cream with the cream cheese and the other ingredients, pulse well, divide into cups and serve cold.

Nutrition: Calories: 254 Fat: 24 g Fiber: 1 g Carbs: 2 g Protein: 8 g

117. SUGAR-FREE LOW CARB COFFEE RICOTTA MOUSSE

Preparation time: 15 minutes - Cooking time: 2 hours - Servings: 10

Ingredients:

- 1½ tsps. Dry gelatin - 1 tsp. vanilla liquid stevia - ½ cup of hot brewed coffee
- Pinch of salt - 2 cups of Ricotta cheese - 1 tsp. vanilla extract - 1 tsp. instant espresso
- Shaved sugar free chocolate to garnish (optional) - 1 cup of heavy whipping cream

Directions:

1. Pour the gelatin into the hot coffee and stir properly until it dissolves.
2. Set it aside and allow it to cool. Add the ricotta, vanilla extract, salt, stevia, and espresso and blend the ingredients until combined.
3. Pour the cooled coffee-gelatin mixture and blend until smooth.
4. Pour in the whipping cream and blend on high until it's thickened and whipped.
5. Spoon into serving dishes then garnish with shaved chocolate if you wish.
6. Keep in the refrigerator for 2 hours and enjoy.

Nutrition: Calories: 170 Fat: 15.2 g Carbohydrates: 2.5 g Protein: 6.9 g Sugar: 2.5 g

118. LEMON-YOGURT MOUSSE

Preparation time: 5 minutes - Cooking time: 1 hour - Servings: 4

Ingredients:

- 24 Oz plain yogurt, strained overnight in cheesecloth - 2 cups swerve confectioner's sugar
- 2 lemons, juiced and zested - Pink salt to taste - 1 cup whipped cream + extra for garnish

Directions:

1. Whip the plain yogurt in a bowl with a hand mixer until light and fluffy.
2. Mix in the sugar, lemon juice, and salt. Fold in the whipped cream to evenly combine.
3. Spoon the mousse into serving cups and refrigerate to thicken for 1 hour.
4. Swirl with extra whipped cream and garnish lightly with lemon zest. Serve immediately.

Nutrition: Calories: 223 Fat: 18 g Net Carbs: 3 g Protein: 12 g

119. BLUEBERRIES MOUSSE

Preparation time: 10 minutes - Cooking time: 20 minutes - Servings: 6

Ingredients:

- 8 ounces heavy cream - 1 teaspoon vanilla extract - 1 tablespoon stevia - 1 cup blueberries

Directions:

1. Combine all ingredients in a blender, pulse well, divide into bowls and serve cold.

Nutrition: Calories 219 Fat: 21.1 g Fiber: 0.9 g Carbs: 7 g Protein: 1.4 g

120. EASY CITRUS MOUSSE WITH ALMONDS

Preparation time: 5 minutes - Cooking time: 1 hour - Servings: 2-4

Ingredients:

- 3/4 lb. cream cheese, softened - 2 cups swerve confectioner's sugar
- 1 lemon, juiced and zested - 1 lime, juice and zested - Salt to taste
- 1 cup whipped cream + extra for garnish - ¼ cup toasted almonds, chopped

Directions:

1. In a bowl and with a hand mixer, whip the cream cheese until light and fluffy. Add in the sugar, lemon and lime juices and salt, and mix well.
2. Fold in the whipped cream to evenly combine.
3. Spoon the mousse into serving cups and refrigerate to thicken for 1 hour. Swirl with extra whipped cream and garnish with lemon and lime zest.
4. Serve immediately topped with almonds.

Nutrition: Calories: 242 Fat: 18 g Net Carbs: 3.3 g Protein: 6.5 g

121. STRAWBERRY CHOCOLATE MOUSSE

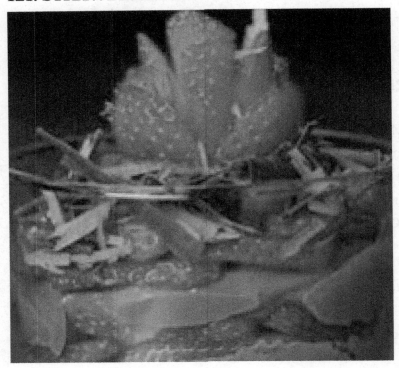

Preparation time: 30 minutes - Cooking time: 30 minutes - Servings: 2

Ingredients:

- 3 eggs
- ½ cup dark chocolate chips
- 1 cup heavy cream
- 1 cup fresh strawberries, sliced
- 1 vanilla extract
- 1 tbsp. xylitol

Directions:

1. Prepare the bowl of chocolate and put it in the microwave for a minute on high and let it cool for 10 minutes.
2. Whip the cream until very soft on a separate bowl.
3. Add the eggs, vanilla extract, and xylitol; whisk to combine. Fold in the cooled chocolate.
4. Divide the mousse between glasses, top with the strawberry slices and chill in the fridge for at least 30 minutes before serving.

Nutrition: Calories: 567 Fat: 45.6 g Net Carbs: 9.6 g Protein: 13.6 g

BARS RECIPES

122. MIXED-NUT GRANOLA BARS

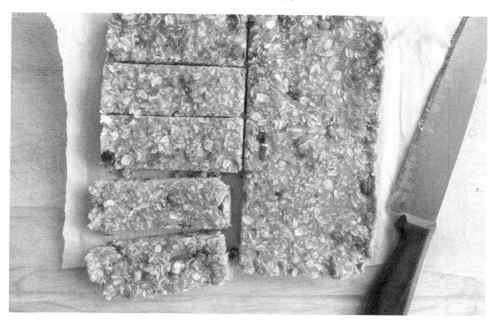

Preparation time: 5 minutes - Cooking time: 20 minutes - Servings: 14

Ingredients

- ½ cup pumpkin seeds - ½ cup sunflower seeds
- ½ cup coarsely chopped almonds - ¼ cup unsweetened shredded coconut
- ¼ cup coconut oil, melted - 4 tbsp. no sugar added almond butter
- 1 tsp. vanilla extract - 2 tsp. ground cinnamon - 1/8 tsp. salt
- 3 tbsp. granular swerve - 2 large eggs

Directions:

1. Preheat the oven to 350F.
2. In a food processor, process almonds and seeds to break them up slightly.
3. Add remaining ingredients and pulse until mixed.
4. Spread mixture into an 8 x 8-inch silicone baking dish.
5. Bake for 20 minutes. Cool, cut, and serve.

Nutrition: Calories: 165 Fat: 14.4 g Carb: 7.8 g Protein: 5.0 g

123. CHOCOLATE CRUNCH BARS

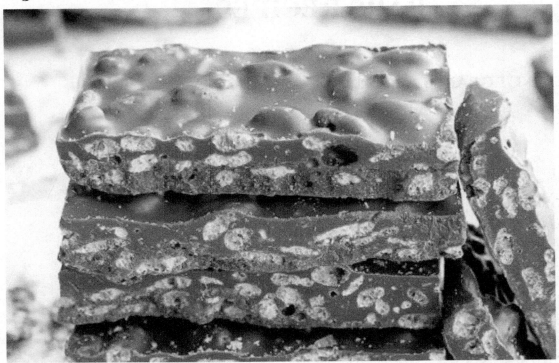

Preparation time: 5 minutes - Cooking time: 5 minutes - Servings: 20

Ingredients

- 1 ½ cups chocolate chips of choice (stevia sweetened)
- 1 cup almond butter
- ½ cup sticky sweetener of choice
- ¼ cup coconut oil
- 3 cups nuts and seeds of choice

Directions:

1. Line an 8 x 8-inch baking dish with parchment paper and set aside.
2. In a pan, combine coconut oil, sticky sweetener, almond butter, and chocolate chips and melt until combined.
3. Add your nuts and seeds of choice and mix until fully combined.
4. Pour the crunch bar mixture into the lined baking dish and spread out using a spatula.
5. Refrigerate until firm. Slice and serve.

Nutrition: Calories: 155 Fat: 12 g Carb: 4 g Protein: 7 g

124. EASY PUMPKIN BAR

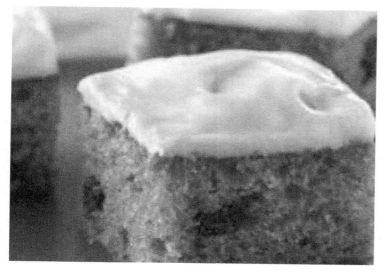

Preparation Time: 10 minutes - Cooking Time: 30 minutes - Servings: 32

Ingredients:

- 5 eggs - 1 cup pumpkin puree - 1 cup olive oil
- 1 tsp baking powder - 1 tsp baking soda
- 2 cups almond flour - 1 cup Swerve - 1/2 tsp sea salt

For frosting:

- 16 oz. cream cheese, softened
- 1 tsp vanilla
- 1 cup Swerve
- 8 tbsp. butter, softened

Directions:

1. For frosting: Add all ingredients into the mixing bowl and beat until smooth. Set aside.
2. Preheat the oven to 350 F. Grease 18*13 baking sheet and set aside.
3. In a large bowl, beat eggs, pumpkin puree, sweetener, and oil using a hand mixer until well combined.
4. In a separate bowl, mix together almond flour, baking powder, baking soda, and salt.
5. Add almond flour mixture into the egg mixture and beat until just combined.
6. Pour batter in a prepared baking sheet and spread evenly and bake for 25-30 minutes.
7. Let it cool completely then spread frosting on top.
8. Slice and serve.

Nutrition: Calories 184 Fat 18.2 g Carbohydrates 2.8 g Sugar 0.4 g Protein 3.6 g Cholesterol 49 mg

125. SWEET & TANGY LEMON BARS

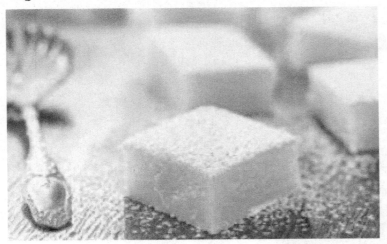

Preparation Time: 10 minutes - Cooking Time: 27 minutes - Servings: 9

Ingredients:

For crust:

- 2 tbsp. Swerve
- 1 1/4 cups almond flour
- 1/2 cup butter, melted

For filling:

- 3 eggs
- 1/3 cup coconut flour
- 3/4 cup Swerve
- 1/3 cup fresh lemon juice

Directions:

1. Add all filling ingredients into the food processor and process until smooth and place in the refrigerator for 20 minutes to thicken.
2. For crust: Preheat the oven to 350 F.
3. Line 8*8-inch pan with parchment paper and set aside.
4. Mix together almond flour, swerve, and butter until well combined.
5. Transfer almond flour mixture into the prepared pan and spread evenly and press down.
6. Bake crust for 7 minutes. Remove from the oven and let it cool.
7. Pour filling over crust and bake for 20 minutes.
8. Let it cool completely then slice and serve.

Nutrition: Calories 226 Fat 19.6 g Carbohydrates 7.2 g Sugar 0.3 g Protein 6 g Cholesterol 82 mg

126. CHOCO CHIP BARS

Preparation Time: 10 minutes - Cooking Time: 20 minutes - Servings: 8

Ingredients:

- 1 stick butter - 2/3 cup unsweetened chocolate chips - 1 tsp vanilla
- 1/2 cup collagen - 1/3 cup Swerve - 1/3 cup coconut flour - 1 cup almond flour

Directions:

1. Preheat the oven to 350 F.
2. Line 8*10-inch cookie sheet with parchment paper and set aside.
3. Add all ingredients except chocolate chips into the food processor and process until fully incorporated.
4. Add chocolate chips and mix well. Transfer mixture onto the prepared cookie sheet and spread evenly and press down.
5. Bake for 20 minutes. Slice and serve.

Nutrition: Calories 342 Fat 29.3 g Carbohydrates 12 g Sugar 0.1 g Protein 6.8 g Cholesterol 30 mg

127. CHOCO CHIPS COCONUT BARS

Preparation Time: 10 minutes - Cooking Time: 30 minutes - Servings: 16

Ingredients:

- 1/2 cup unsweetened chocolate chips - 2 eggs, lightly beaten
- 1 1/2 tsp vanilla - 1/2 cup almond milk - 1/2 cup Swerve
- 1/2 cup butter, melted - 1/2 tsp baking powder
- 1/2 cup unsweetened shredded coconut
- 1/4 cup coconut flour - 3/4 cup almond flour

Directions:

1. Preheat the oven to 350 F.
2. Line 8*8-inch baking pan with parchment paper and set aside.
3. In a medium bowl, mix together almond flour, baking powder, shredded coconut, and coconut flour.
4. In a separate bowl, whisk eggs, vanilla, almond milk, sweetener, and butter.
5. Pour egg mixture into the almond flour mixture and mix until well combined.
6. Add chocolate chips and mix well.
7. Spread mixture into the prepared baking pan and bake for 25-30 minutes.
8. Slice and serve.

Nutrition: Calories 156 Fat 16.8 g Carbohydrates 5.8 g Sugar 0.6 g Protein 3.5 g Cholesterol 36 mg

128. WHITE CHOCOLATE PEANUT BUTTER BARS

Preparation Time: 10 minutes - Cooking Time: 25 minutes - Servings: 16

Ingredients:

- 2 eggs - 1/4 cup cocoa butter, chopped - 1/2 cup Swerve
- 1 tbsp. coconut flour - 1/4 cup almond flour - 3 tbsp. cocoa butter, melted
- 1 tsp vanilla - 4 tbsp. butter, softened - 1/2 cup peanut butter

Directions:

1. Preheat the oven to 350 F.
2. Line 9*9-inch baking pan with parchment paper and set aside.
3. In a mixing bowl, beat peanut butter, butter, eggs, vanilla, and melted cocoa butter until smooth.
4. Add flours, sweetener, and chopped cocoa butter and mix well.
5. Spread peanut butter mixture in the prepared baking pan and bake for 25 minutes.
6. Let it cool completely then place in the refrigerator for 2 hours.
7. Slice and serve.

Nutrition: Calories 108 Fat 9.9 g Carbohydrates 2.4 g Sugar 0.8 g Protein 3.2 g Cholesterol 28 mg

129. HEALTHY PUMPKIN BARS

Preparation Time: 10 minutes Cooking Time: 30 minutes Servings: 16

Ingredients:

- 2 eggs - 1 tsp baking soda - 1 1/2 tsp pumpkin pie spice
- 1 1/2 cups almond flour - 1 tsp vanilla - 1/4 cup Swerve
- 2 tbsp. avocado oil - 1/2 cup pumpkin puree - 1/2 tsp salt

Directions:

1. Preheat the oven to 350 F.
2. Line 8*8-inch baking pan with parchment paper and set aside.
3. In a medium bowl, mix together pumpkin, eggs, sweetener, vanilla, and oil until well combined.
4. Add almond flour, baking soda, pumpkin spice, and salt and mix well.
5. Pour batter into the prepared pan and bake for 25-30 minutes.
6. Slice and serve.

Nutrition: Calories 77 Fat 5.8 g Carbohydrates 3.2 g Sugar 0.3 g Protein 3.1 g Cholesterol 20 mg

130. MOIST LEMON BARS

Preparation Time: 10 minutes - Cooking Time: 40 minutes - Servings: 8

Ingredients:

- 4 eggs - 1/3 cup erythritol - 2 tsp baking powder - 2 cups almond flour
- 1 lemon zest - 1/4 cup fresh lemon juice - 1/2 cup butter, softened - 1/2 cup sour cream

Directions:

1. Preheat the oven to 350 F.
2. Line 9*6-inch baking pan with parchment paper and set aside.
3. In a mixing bowl, beat eggs until frothy.
4. Add butter and sour cream and beat until well combined.
5. Add remaining ingredients and blend everything well until fully incorporated.
6. Pour batter into the prepared baking pan and bake for 35-40 minutes.
7. Let it cool completely then slice and serve.

Nutrition: Calories 335 Fat 30 g Carbohydrates 7.6 g Sugar 0.4 g Protein 9.4 g Cholesterol 119 mg

131. PEANUT BUTTER PROTEIN BARS

Preparation Time: 10 minutes - Cooking Time: 25 minutes - Servings: 8

Ingredients:

For first layer:

- 1 1/2 tbsp. swerve - 1 tbsp. protein powder
- 1 1/2 tbsp. coconut flour - 1/2 cup peanut butter

For second layer:

- 1 1/2 tbsp. coconut flour - 1 tbsp. protein powder - 1 1/2 tbsp. swerve
- 1 tbsp. unsweetened cocoa powder - 1/2 cup peanut butter

Directions:

1. Preheat the oven to 350 F.
2. Line baking pan with parchment paper and set aside.
3. In a mixing bowl, mix together first layer ingredients until well combined and spread into the prepared baking pan.
4. In a separate bowl, mix together second layer ingredients until combined. Spread on top of first layer.
5. Bake for 25 minutes.
6. Let it cool completely then slice and serve.

Nutrition: Calories 207 Fat 16.7 g Carbohydrates 9.5 g Sugar 3.1 g Protein 9 g Cholesterol 1 mg

132. ALMOND CHOCOLATE BARS

Preparation Time: 10 minutes - Cooking Time: 10 minutes - Servings: 8

Ingredients:

- 1/2 cup almonds, chopped - 1/2 tsp vanilla - 3 tbsp. Swerve - 1/2 cup coconut oil
- 2 tbsp. unsweetened cocoa powder - 1/4 cup unsweetened chocolate chips

Directions:

1. Add chocolate chips and coconut oil in a microwave-safe bowl and microwave for 30 seconds or until chocolate and oil are melted. Stir well.
2. Add cocoa powder and sweetener into the melted chocolate and mix until smooth.
3. Add vanilla and stir well.
4. Pour chocolate mixture onto the wax paper-lined baking sheet.
5. Sprinkle chopped almonds on top of chocolate mixture.
6. Place the baking sheet in the refrigerator for 2 hours.
7. Cut into pieces and serve.

Nutrition: Calories 208 Fat 20.8 g Carbohydrates 4.8 g Sugar 0.3 g Protein 2.5 g Cholesterol 0 mg

133. APPLE PIE BARS

Preparation Time: 10 minutes - Cooking Time: 10 minutes - Servings: 12

Ingredients:

- 1/2 cup unsweetened applesauce - 1/2 cup Swerve
- 1/4 cup almond butter - 1 tsp nutmeg
- 1 tsp mixed spice
- 1 tbsp. cinnamon
- 1/2 cup protein powder
- 1/2 cup almond flour
- 1 cup coconut flour

Directions:

1. Line baking dish with parchment paper and set aside.
2. Add almond butter in microwave-safe bowl and microwave until butter is melted.
3. In a mixing bowl, mix together all ingredients until well combined.
4. Transfer mixture into the prepared baking dish and spread evenly press firmly.
5. Place baking dish in the refrigerator for 30 minutes.
6. Slice and serve.

Nutrition: Calories 92 Fat 3.7 g Carbohydrates 10 g Sugar 1.2 g Protein 5.3 g Cholesterol 8 mg

134. CHOCOLATE CHEESECAKE BARS

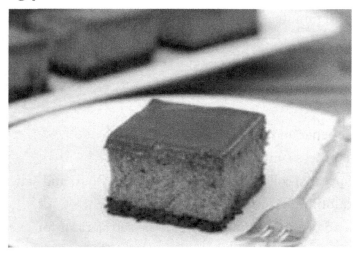

Preparation Time: 10 minutes - Cooking Time: 10 minutes - Servings: 12

Ingredients:

For crust:

- 1 tsp vanilla
- 1/3 cup butter, melted
- 1 tsp stevia
- 3 tbsp. unsweetened cocoa powder
- 1 3/4 cup almond flour

For filling:

- 1 tsp stevia
- 1 tsp vanilla
- 15 oz. cream cheese
- 10 oz. unsweetened chocolate, melted

Directions:

1. Line 7*7-inch pan with parchment paper and set aside.
2. In a mixing bowl, mix together all crust ingredients and spread evenly into the prepared pan.
3. For the filling: Add all filling ingredients into the medium bowl and beat until well combined.
4. Pour filling mixture over crust and spread well. Place pan in the fridge for 2 hours or until set. Slice and serve.

Nutrition: Calories 390 Fat 38 g Carbohydrates 12.3 g Sugar 0.4 g Protein 9.5 g Cholesterol 53 mg

135. PECAN PIE BARS

Preparation Time: 10 minutes - Cooking Time: 10 minutes - Servings: 10

Ingredients:

- 1 1/2 cups pecans, toasted - 1 tsp vanilla - 6 tbsp. butter, melted
- 1/4 cup collagen - 6 tbsp. Swerve - 1 cup almond flour - 1/2 tsp salt

Directions:

1. Line 8-inch baking pan with parchment paper and set aside.
2. Add pecans into the food processor and process until course.
3. In a mixing bowl, mix together ground pecans, collagen, sweetener, almond flour, and salt.
4. Add vanilla and melted butter and mix until well combined.
5. Spread mixture into the prepared pan and press firmly and place in the refrigerator for 1 hour. Slice and serve.

Nutrition: Calories 265 Fat 25.8 g Carbohydrates 6.4 g Sugar 0.7 g Protein 4.7 g Cholesterol 18 mg

136. BUTTER BARS

Preparation Time: 10 minutes - Cooking Time: 20 minutes - Servings: 9

Ingredients:

- 1/2 cup butter, melted
- 1/3 cup walnuts, chopped
- 1 tbsp. psyllium husk powder
- 2 cups almond flour
- 1 tsp vanilla
- 1 egg, lightly beaten
- 1/2 tsp baking powder
- 1/2 cup Swerve
- 1/4 tsp salt

Directions:

1. Preheat the oven to 375 F. Line 9*9-inch pan with parchment paper and set aside.
2. Add all ingredients except walnuts into the mixing bowl and mix until well combined.
3. Add walnuts and stir well.
4. Pour batter into the prepared pan and bake for 20 minutes.
5. Let it cool completely then slice and serve.

Nutrition: Calories 281 Fat 25.3 g Carbohydrates 7 g Sugar 0.2 g Protein 7.2 g Cholesterol 45 mg

137. EASY COCONUT BARS

Preparation Time: 10 minutes - Cooking Time: 10 minutes - Servings: 20

Ingredients:

- 3 cups unsweetened shredded coconut - 3/4 cup Swerve
- 1/3 cup coconut oil - 1 tbsp. lemon rind, chopped

Directions:

1. Line 8*8-inch pan with parchment paper and set aside.
2. Add all ingredients into the large bowl and mix until well combined.
3. Pour batter into the prepared pan and spread evenly and place in freezer until firm.
4. Slice and serve.

Nutrition: Calories 133 Fat 13.3 g Carbohydrates 3.9 g Sugar 1.1 g Protein 1.1 g Cholesterol 0 mg

138. NUT BUTTER PROTEIN BARS

Preparation Time: 10 minutes - Cooking Time: 10 minutes - Servings: 12

Ingredients:

- 1 cup almond butter - 10 drops liquid stevia - 2 scoops vanilla protein powder
- 4 tbsp. coconut oil, melted - 1/2 tsp salt

Directions:

1. Line baking pan with parchment paper and set aside.
2. Add all ingredients into the mixing bowl and mix until well combined.
3. Pour mixture into the prepared pan and spread evenly and place in the fridge until firm.
4. Slice and serve.

Nutrition: Calories 66 Fat 5.3 g Carbohydrates 0.3 g Sugar 0.1 g Protein 4.8 g Cholesterol 0 mg

139. WHITE CHOCOLATE BARS

Preparation Time: 10 minutes - Cooking Time: 10 minutes - Servings: 12

Ingredients:

- 2 oz. cocoa butter, chopped - 1 tsp pumpkin seeds, toasted
- 1/2 tsp hemp seed powder - 1 tsp vanilla - 1/3 cup swerve - Pinch of salt

Directions:

1. Add cocoa butter into the medium bowl and melt butter in a double boiler.
2. Add remaining ingredients into the melted cocoa butter and mix well.
3. Pour mixture into the greased baking pan and place it in the refrigerator for 1 hour.
4. Cut into pieces and serve.

Nutrition: Calories 46 Fat 4.9 g Carbohydrates 0.2 g Sugar 0 g Protein 0.1 g Cholesterol 0 mg

140. EASY PEANUT BUTTER BARS

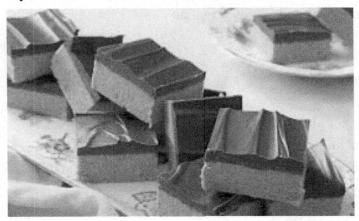

Preparation Time: 10 minutes - Cooking Time: 10 minutes - Servings: 8

Ingredients:

For crust:

- 1 tbsp. Swerve
- 1/2 tsp cinnamon
- 1/4 cup butter, melted
- 1 cup almond flour
- Pinch of salt

For filling:

- 1/4 cup heavy cream
- 1/8 tsp xanthan gum
- 1/2 tsp vanilla
- 1/4 cup Swerve
- 1/2 cup peanut butter
- 1/4 cup butter, melted

Directions:

1. Line baking pan with parchment paper and set aside.
2. Mix together all crust ingredients and spread into the prepared pan.
3. Bake crust for 10 minutes at 350 F.
4. In a mixing bowl, add all filling ingredients and beat until just combined.
5. Once the crust is cool then spread filling on top of crust and place in freezer for 2 hours.
6. Slice and serve.

Nutrition: Calories 295 Fat 27.7 g Carbohydrates 6.8 g Sugar 1.5 g Protein 7.2 g Cholesterol 36 mg

141. COCONUT BLUEBERRY BARS

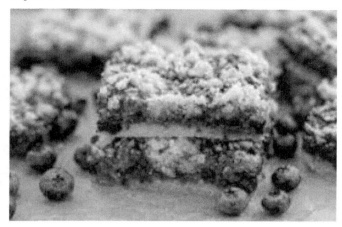

Preparation Time: 10 minutes - Cooking Time: 50 minutes - Servings: 4

Ingredients:

- 1/4 cup coconut flakes
- 3 tbsp. coconut oil
- 2 tbsp. coconut flour
- 1/2 cup almond flour
- 3 tbsp. water
- 1 tbsp. chia seeds
- 1/4 cup blueberries
- 1 tsp vanilla
- 1 tsp fresh lemon juice
- 2 tbsp. erythritol
- 1/4 cup almonds, sliced

Directions:

1. Preheat the oven to 300 F.
2. Line baking dish with parchment paper and set aside.
3. In a small bowl, mix water and chia seeds. Set aside.
4. In a mixing bowl, combine together all ingredients. Add chia mixture and stir well.
5. Pour mixture into the prepared dish and spread evenly and bake for 50 minutes.
6. Slice and serve.

Nutrition: Calories 264 Fat 23.1 g Carbohydrates 9.2 g Sugar 1.7 g Protein 5.8 g Cholesterol 0 mg

PIES AND TARTS RECIPES

142. PEANUT BUTTER PIE

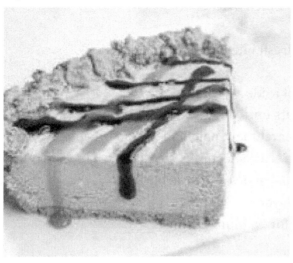

Servings: 16 - Preparation time: 15 minutes - Cooking time: 10 minutes

Ingredients:

For crust:

- 3/4 cup almond flour - ½ cup of cocoa powder - ½ cup erythritol
- 1/3 cup almond butter - ½ cup butter softened

For filling:

- 1 ½ cups heavy whipping cream - ½ cup erythritol
- 1/3 cup peanut butter - 8 oz. cream cheese, softened

Directions:

1. For the crust: In a large bowl, combine together butter, cocoa powder, sweetener, and almond butter until smooth. Add almond flour and beat until mixture stiff.

2. Transfer crust mixture into the greased spring-form cake pan and spread evenly and place in the refrigerator for 15-30 minutes.

3. Meanwhile for filling: In a mixing bowl, beat sweetener, peanut butter, and cream cheese until smooth. Add heavy cream and beat until stiff peaks form.

4. Spread filling mixture in prepared crust and refrigerate for 2 hours. Slice and serve.

Nutrition: Net Carbs: 2.7 g; Calories: 209; Total Fat: 20.7 g; Saturated Fat: 10.3 g Protein: 4.4 g; Carbs: 4.4 g; Fiber: 1.7 g; Sugar: 0.8 g; Fat 88% Protein 7% Carbs 5%

143. DELICIOUS BLUEBERRY PIE

Preparation time: 10 minutes - Cooking time: 25 minutes - Servings: 8

Ingredients:

For crust:

- 4 eggs - 1 tbsp. water - ¼ tsp baking powder
- 1 ½ cups coconut flour - 1 cup butter, melted - Pinch of salt

For filling:

- 8 oz. cream cheese - 2 tbsp. swerve - 1 ½ cup fresh blueberries

Directions:

1. Spray 9-inch pie pan with cooking spray and set aside.
2. In a large bowl, mix together all crust ingredients until dough is formed.
3. Divide dough in half and roll out between two parchment paper sheet and set aside.
4. Preheat the oven to 350 F/ 180 C. Transfer one crust sheet into greased pie pan.
5. Spread cream cheese on crust. Mix together blueberries and sweetener.
6. Spread blueberries on top of the cream cheese layer.
7. Cover pie with other half rolled crust and bake for 25 minutes.
8. Allow to cool completely then slice and serve.

Nutrition: Net Carbs: 5.4 g; Calories: 362 Total Fat: 35.6 g; Saturated Fat: 21.9 g Protein: 5.7 g; Carbs: 7 g; Fiber: 1.6 g; Sugar: 3.1 g; Fat 88% Protein 6% Carbs 6%

144. QUICK & SIMPLE STRAWBERRY TART

Preparation time: 10 minutes - Cooking time: 22 minutes - Servings: 10

Ingredients:

- 5 egg whites - ½ cup butter, melted - 1 tsp baking powder
- 1 tsp vanilla - 1 lemon zest, grated - 1 ½ cup almond flour - 1/3 cup xylitol

Directions:

1. Preheat the oven to 375 F/ 190 C.
2. Spray the tart pan with cooking spray and set aside.
3. In a bowl, whisk egg whites until foamy.
4. Add sweetener and whisk until soft peaks form.
5. Add remaining ingredients except for strawberries and fold until well combined.
6. Pour mixture into the prepared tart pan and top with sliced strawberries.
7. Bake in preheated oven for 20-22 minutes. Serve and enjoy.

Nutrition: Net Carbs: 3.9 g; Calories: 195; Total Fat: 17.7 g; Saturated Fat: 6.4 g Protein: 5.6 g; Carbs: 5.9 g; Fiber: 2 g; Sugar: 0.9 g; Fat 81% Protein 11% Carbs 8%

145. DELICIOUS CUSTARD TARTS

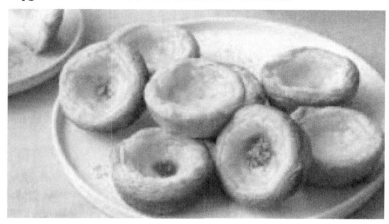

Preparation time: 10 minutes - Cooking time: 30 minutes - Servings: 8

Ingredients:

For crust:

- 3/4 cup coconut flour - 1 tbsp. swerve - 2 eggs
- ½ cup of coconut oil - Pinch of salt

For custard:

- 3 eggs - ½ tsp nutmeg - 5 tbsp. swerve
- 1 ½ tsp vanilla - 1 ¼ cup unsweetened almond milk

Directions:

1. For the crust: Preheat the oven to 400 F/ 200 C.
2. In a bowl, beat eggs, coconut oil, sweetener, and salt.
3. Add coconut flour and mix until dough is formed.
4. Add dough in the tart pan and spread evenly.
5. Prick dough with a knife. Bake in preheated oven for 10 minutes.
6. For the custard: Heat almond milk and vanilla in a small pot until simmering.
7. Whisk together eggs and sweetener in a bowl.
8. Slowly add almond milk and whisk constantly.
9. Strain custard well and pour into baked tart base.
10. Bake in the oven at 300 F for 30 minutes. Sprinkle nutmeg on top and serve.

Nutrition: Net Carbs: 2.2 g; Calories: 175; Total Fat: 17.2 g; Saturated Fat: 12.9 g Protein: 3.8 g; Carbs: 2.9 g; Fiber: 0.7 g; Sugar: 0.4 g; Fat 87% Protein 8% Carbs 5%

146. CHOCOLATE PIE

Preparation Time: 10 minutes - Cooking Time: 25 minutes - Servings: 8

Ingredients:

- 4 eggs - 1 tsp baking powder - 2 tbsp. coconut flour
- 1 cup unsweetened cocoa powder - 1 tbsp. vanilla - 2 tsp liquid stevia
- 1 1/3 cup unsweetened coconut milk - 1/4 tsp kosher salt

Directions:

1. Preheat the oven to 325 F.
2. Grease 9-inch pie dish and set aside.
3. In a large bowl, whisk together eggs, vanilla, sweetener, and coconut milk.
4. Add cocoa powder, coconut flour, and salt and whisk until well combined.
5. Pour mixture into the prepared dish and bake for 25 minutes.
6. Let it cool completely then place in freezer for 2 hours.
7. Slice and serve.

Nutrition: Calories 161 Fat 13.5 g Carbohydrates 9.7 g Sugar 2 g Protein 6.1 g Cholesterol 82 mg

147. PUMPKIN CHEESE PIE

Preparation Time: 10 minutes - Cooking Time: 55 minutes - Servings: 8

Ingredients:

- 2 eggs - 1 tsp vanilla - 1 tbsp. pumpkin pie spice
- 1 tsp lemon juice - 8 oz. mascarpone cheese
- 1/2 cup Swerve - 1 cup pumpkin puree

Directions:

1. Preheat the oven to 350 F.
2. In a bowl, beat pumpkin puree and sweetener.
3. Add eggs and blend well.
4. Add lemon juice, vanilla, and spices and blend well.
5. Add cheese and blend until smooth.
6. Pour batter into the greased pie dish and bake for 55 minutes.
7. Let it cool completely then place in freezer for 2 hours.
8. Slice and serve.

Nutrition: Calories 80 Fat 5 g Carbohydrates 4.1 g Sugar 1.3 g Protein 5 g Cholesterol 55 mg

148. EASY & DELICIOUS PECAN PIE

Preparation Time: 10 minutes - Cooking Time: 20 minutes - Servings: 8

Ingredients:

- 1/2 tsp cinnamon
- 1/2 tsp vanilla
- 1 cup pecan, crushed
- 1/4 cup ground flax seed+ 1/2 cup water
- 1/2 cup erythritol
- 1/2 cup coconut milk

Directions:

1. Preheat the oven to 400 F.
2. Line 9-inch pie pan with parchment paper and set aside.
3. In a small bowl, mix together flaxseed and water and set aside for 5 minutes.
4. In a mixing bowl, add all ingredients and mix until fully combined.
5. Pour mixture into the prepared pie pan and bake for 20 minutes.
6. Let it cool completely. Slice and serve.

Nutrition: Calories 158 Fat 15 g Carbohydrates 4.8 g Sugar 1 g Protein 2.7 g Cholesterol 0 mg

149. MINI PUMPKIN PIE

Preparation Time: 10 minutes - Cooking Time: 60 minutes - Servings: 6

Ingredients:

- 2 eggs - 1/2 tsp vanilla - 1/2 tsp cinnamon
- 1 1/2 tsp pumpkin pie spice - 1/2 cup Swerve
- 1 cup unsweetened almond milk - 15 oz. pumpkin puree

Directions:

1. Preheat the oven to 425 F. In a mixing bowl, whisk eggs.
2. Add vanilla, spices, sweetener, almond milk, and pumpkin and whisk until smooth.
3. Divide mixture evenly into the 6 ramekins and bake for 15 minutes.
4. Turn temperature to 350 F and bake for 45 minutes more.
5. Let it cool completely then place in freezer for 2 hours.
6. Serve and enjoy.

Nutrition: Calories 55 Fat 2.3 g Carbohydrates 6.8 g Sugar 2.5 g Protein 2.8 g Cholesterol 55 mg

150. EASY CRUSTLESS PUMPKIN PIE

Preparation Time: 10 minutes - Cooking Time: 45 minutes - Servings: 8

Ingredients:

- 15 oz. can pumpkin puree - 2 eggs - 1 tsp pumpkin pie spice
- 1/2 tsp vanilla - 1/2 tsp nutmeg - 1 tsp cinnamon
- 1/3 cup Swerve - 8 oz. unsweetened almond milk

Directions:

1. Preheat the oven to 375 F.
2. Grease 9-inch pie pan and set aside.
3. Add all ingredients into the mixing bowl and beat until smooth and well combined.
4. Pour batter into the prepared pan and bake for 40-45 minutes.
5. Let it cool completely.
6. Slice and serve.

Nutrition: Calories 46 Fat 1.6 g Carbohydrates 5.7 g Sugar 2 g Protein 2.4 g Cholesterol 41 mg

151. FLAVORFUL CUSTARD PIE

Preparation Time: 10 minutes - Cooking Time: 45 minutes - Servings: 8

Ingredients:

- 2 eggs - 4 oz. unsweetened shredded coconut
- 1/2 tsp lemon extract - 1 tsp lemon zest
- 3/4 tsp baking powder - 1 tsp vanilla
- 2 tbsp. butter, melted - 1/4 cup coconut flour
- 3/4 cup Swerve - 1 cup unsweetened coconut milk

Directions:

1. Preheat the oven to 350 F.
2. Grease 9-inch pie pan and set aside.
3. In a large bowl, add all ingredients except shredded coconut and beat until well combined.
4. Add shredded coconut and fold well.
5. Pour batter into the prepared pie pan and bake for 40-45 minutes.
6. Let it cool completely.
7. Slice and serve.

Nutrition: Calories 287 Fat 27.4 g Carbohydrates 8.3 g Sugar 2.5 g Protein 3.6 g Cholesterol 41 mg

152. COCONUT PUMPKIN PIE

Preparation Time: 10 minutes - Cooking Time: 45 minutes - Servings: 8

Ingredients:

- 3 eggs - 2 tbsp. coconut flour
- 1 cup unsweetened coconut milk
- 1 tbsp. vanilla
- 1 tbsp. pumpkin pie spice
- 1 1/2 tsp liquid stevia
- 15 oz. can pumpkin puree

Directions:

1. Preheat the oven to 350 F.
2. Grease 9-inch pie pan and set aside.
3. In a mixing bowl, whisk eggs, vanilla, pumpkin pie spice, stevia, and pumpkin puree.
4. Add remaining ingredients and stir until well combined.
5. Pour batter into the prepared pie pan and bake for 40-45 minutes.
6. Let it cool completely then place in freezer for 2 hours.
7. Serve and enjoy.

Nutrition: Calories 129 Fat 9.1 g Carbohydrates 8.4 g Sugar 3.3 g Protein 4 g Cholesterol 61 mg

153. PERFECT MINI PUMPKIN PIE

Preparation Time: 10 minutes - Cooking Time: 40 minutes - Servings: 12

Ingredients:

- 2 eggs - 1/2 cup lakanto monk fruit
- 2 1/2 tbsp. pumpkin pie spice
- 1 cup heavy cream
- 1 3/4 cup pumpkin puree - 1/4 tsp salt

Directions:

1. Add all ingredients into the mixing bowl and mix until well combined.
2. Pour batter into the 12 muffin molds and bake at 425 F for 10 minutes.
3. After 10 minutes turn temperature to 350 F and bake for 30 minutes.
4. Let it cool completely.
5. Serve and enjoy.

Nutrition: Calories 71 Fat 4.7 g Carbohydrates 6 g Sugar 3.3 g Protein 1.6 g Cholesterol 41 mg

154. STRAWBERRY CHEESE PIE

Preparation Time: 10 minutes - Cooking Time: 10 minutes - Servings: 10

Ingredients:

- 1 cup almond flour - 1/2 cup erythritol - 1/2 cup fresh strawberries
- 1/4 cup strawberries, chopped - 3/4 cup heavy whipping cream
- 1/4 cup butter, melted - 8 oz. cream cheese, softened

Directions:

1. In a bowl, mix together almond flour and melted butter.
2. Spread almond flour mixture into the pie dish.
3. Add strawberries in a blender and blend until a smooth puree is formed.
4. Add strawberry puree in a large bowl.
5. Add remaining ingredients except for chopped strawberries and whisk until thick.
6. Add chopped strawberries and fold well.
7. Transfer filling mixture on top of the crust and spread evenly.
8. Place in refrigerator for 2 hours. Slice and serve.

Nutrition: Calories 226 Fat 21.9 g Carbohydrates 3.7 g Sugar 1 g Protein 2 g Cholesterol 49 mg

155. CHEESE TART

Preparation Time: 10 minutes - Cooking Time: 20 minutes - Servings: 10

Ingredients:

For crust:

- 1 egg - 1/2 tsp vanilla - 1/4 cup Swerve - 1/4 cup butter, melted - 2 cups almond flour

For filling:

- 2 tbsp. heavy cream - 1/4 cup Swerve - 3/4 cup lemon curd - 6 oz. mascarpone cheese

Directions:

1. Grease tart pan and set aside. Preheat the oven to 350 F.
2. Add almond flour, vanilla, swerve, egg, and butter into the food processor and process until dough forms.
3. Add the dough into the prepared tart pan and spread out evenly.
4. Prick the crust with a fork and cover with parchment paper and dried beans.
5. Bake for 15 minutes. Remove from the oven and let it cool completely.
6. Add lemon curd, heavy cream, swerve, and mascarpone into the food processor and process until smooth.
7. Pour filling mixture over the crust and spread evenly.
8. Place in refrigerator for 2 hours. Slice and serve.

Nutrition: Calories 304 Fat 27.6 g Carbohydrates 9.6 g Sugar 5.7 g Protein 4 g Cholesterol 101 mg

156. DELICIOUS COCONUT PIE

Preparation Time: 10 minutes - Cooking Time: 20 minutes - Servings: 8

Ingredients:

- 2 oz. shredded coconut - x5.5 oz. coconut flakes - 1 tsp xanthan gum
- 3/4 cup erythritol - 2 cups heavy cream - 6 oz. mascarpone cheese

Directions:

1. Add coconut flakes, erythritol, and coconut oil into the food processor and process for 30 seconds. Transfer coconut mixture into the pie pan. Spread evenly and press firmly.
2. Bake at 350 F for 10 minutes. Heat heavy cream in a saucepan over low heat. Stir in shredded coconut, powdered erythritol, and xanthan gum. Bring to boil.
3. Remove from heat and set aside to cool for 10 minutes.
4. Pour filling mixture over crust and place in the freezer overnight. Slice and serve.

Nutrition: Calories 174 Fat 16.8 g Carbohydrates 3.5 g Sugar 1.2 g Protein 3.4 g Cholesterol 52 mg

157. APPLE CINNAMON TART

Preparation Time: 10 minutes - Cooking Time: 55 minutes - Servings: 10

Ingredients:

For crust:

- 2 cups almond flour - 1/3 cup erythritol - 6 tbsp. butter, melted - 1/2 tsp cinnamon

For filling:

- 3 cups apples, peeled, cored, and sliced - 1/2 tsp cinnamon
- 1/4 cup butter - 1/2 tsp lemon juice - 1/4 cup erythritol

Directions:

1. Preheat the oven to 375 F.
2. For crust: In a bowl, mix together butter, cinnamon, swerve, and almond flour.
3. Transfer crust mixture into the 10-inch springform pan and spread evenly and press firmly. Bake crust for 5 minutes.
4. For filling: In a bowl, mix together apple slices and lemon juice.
5. Arrange apple slices evenly across the bottom of the crust in a circular shape. Press apple slices down gently.
6. In a small bowl, mix together butter, swerve, and cinnamon and microwave for 1 minute.
7. Whisk until smooth and pour over apple slices. Bake tart for 30 minutes.
8. Remove from oven and gently press down apple slices with a fork.
9. Turn heat to 350 F and bake for 20 minutes more. Let it cool completely. Slice and serve.

Nutrition: Calories 281 Fat 23.6 g Carbohydrates 13.5g Sugar 7.8 g Protein 0.3 g Cholesterol 31 mg

158. PECAN LEMON PIE

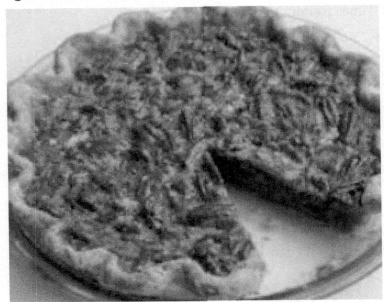

Preparation Time: 10 minutes - Cooking Time: 15 minutes - Servings: 8

Ingredients:

For crust:

- 1 tsp swerve - 2 tbsp. butter, melted - 1 cup pecans, chopped

For filling:

- 1 tsp vanilla - 2/3 cup Swerve - 1/4 cup fresh lemon juice
- 1 tbsp. lemon zest - 1 1/2 cup heavy whipping cream - 8 oz. cream cheese, softened

Directions:

1. Preheat the oven to 350 F. Grease pie pan and set aside.
2. Add pecans into the food processor and process until pecans crushed.
3. Add Swerve and butter into the crushed pecans and mix until combined.
4. Add crust mixture into the prepared pan. Spread evenly and press firmly.
5. Bake crust for 10 minutes. Remove from the oven and let it cool completely.
6. For filling: In a large bowl, beat whipping cream until stiff peaks form.
7. Add remaining filling ingredients and beat until just combined.
8. Pour filling mixture over baked crust and spread evenly.
9. Place in refrigerator for 2 hours. Slice and serve.

Nutrition: Calories 294 Fat 30.1 g Carbohydrates 4 g Sugar 0.8 g Protein 4.1 g Cholesterol 70 mg

159. EASY CRUST-LESS PUMPKIN PIE

Preparation Time: 10 minutes - Cooking Time: 30 minutes - Servings: 4

Ingredients:

- 3 eggs - 1/2 cup pumpkin puree - 1/2 tsp cinnamon - 1 tsp vanilla
- 1/4 cup Swerve - 1/2 cup cream - 1/2 cup unsweetened almond milk

Directions:

1. Preheat the oven to 350 F.
2. Grease square baking dish and set aside.
3. In a large bowl, add all ingredients and whisk until smooth.
4. Pour pie mixture into the prepared dish and bake for 30 minutes.
5. Remove from the oven and let it cool completely.
6. Place into the refrigerator for 2 hours.
7. Slice and serve.

Nutrition: Calories 86 Fat 5.5 g Carbohydrates 4.4 g Sugar 2 g Protein 4.9 g Cholesterol 128 mg

160. CREAM CHEESE BUTTER PIE

Preparation Time: 10 minutes - Cooking Time: 50 minutes - Servings: 8

Ingredients:

For crust:

- 1 egg - 1 1/4 cup almond flour - 1/4 cup butter, melted - 3 tbsp. erythritol

For filling:

- 1 egg - 1 egg yolk - 1 cup butter, melted - 1/2 cup erythritol - 8 oz. cream cheese, softened

Directions:

1. Preheat the oven to 375 F. Grease 9-inch pie dish and set aside.
2. For crust: In a large bowl, mix together all crust ingredients until well combined.
3. Transfer crust mixture into the prepared dish. Spread evenly and press firmly.
4. Bake crust for 7 minutes. Remove from the oven and let it cool completely.
5. For filling: In a mixing bowl, add all filling ingredients and beat until combined.
6. Pour filling mixture over crust and bake at 350 F for 35-40 minutes.
7. Remove from the oven and let it cool completely.
8. Place into the refrigerator for 2 hours.
9. Slice and serve.

Nutrition: Calories 488 Fat 49.7 g Carbohydrates 4 g Sugar 0.8 g Protein 4.2 g Cholesterol 175 mg

161. DELICIOUS STRAWBERRY TART

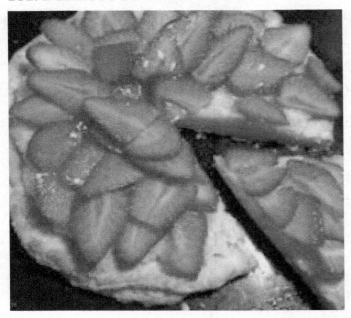

Preparation Time: 10 minutes - Cooking Time: 25 minutes - Servings: 10

Ingredients:

For crust:

- 1 egg - 1 tsp vanilla - 1/4 cup Swerve - 1/4 cup butter, melted - 2 cups almond flour

For filling:

- 6 tbsp. swerve - 8 oz. mascarpone cheese - 1/2 tsp xanthan gum - 1 tsp vanilla
- 4 oz. cream cheese - 1 cup fresh strawberries, sliced - 2 tbsp. heavy cream

Directions:

1. Preheat the oven to 350 F. Grease tart pans and set aside.
2. For crust: Add almond flour, vanilla, swerve, egg, and butter into the food processor and process until dough forms.
3. Transfer dough into the prepared tart pan. Spread dough evenly and press firmly.
4. Prick crust dough with a knife and cover with parchment paper and dried beans.
5. Bake crust for 20 minutes. Remove from the oven and let it cool completely.
6. For filling: Add strawberries, heavy cream, swerve, vanilla, cream cheese, and mascarpone cheese into the food processor and process until smooth. Add xanthan gum and stir well.
7. Pour filling mixture over crust and spread evenly.
8. Place into the refrigerator for 2 hours. Slice and serve.

Nutrition: Calories 291 Fat 25.1 g Carbohydrates 7.6 g Sugar 1.7 g Protein 4.2 g Cholesterol 57 mg

FROZEN RECIPES

162. RASPBERRY SORBET

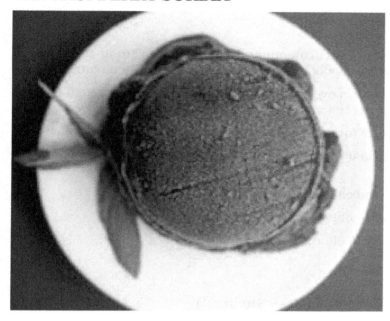

Preparation Time: 15 minutes - Cooking Time: 10 minute - Servings: 8

Ingredients:

- 1 ½ cups raspberries
- 1/4 cup erythritol sweetener
- 2 tablespoons gelatin
- 1 cup water

Directions:

1. Place all the ingredients in a blender and puree until smooth.
2. Pass the mixture through a strainer into a freezer bag, about 1 quart, and place in freezer for 4 hours until thickened, massaging every hour.
3. Then freeze for 6 to 8 hours or until completely firm.
4. When ready to serve, remove the bag from the freezer, thaw for 10 minutes at room temperature and then scoop into serving bowls.

Nutrition: Calories: 43 Cal Carbs: 5 g Fat: 0 g Protein: 1 g Fiber: 3 g

163. SAFFRON PANNACOTTA

Preparation Time: 15 minutes - Cooking Time: 0 minutes - Servings: 6

Ingredients:

- ½ tablespoon gelatin - 1 tablespoon swerve sweetener
- ¼ teaspoon vanilla extract, unsweetened - 1/16 teaspoon saffron
- 2 cups heavy whipping cream, full-fat - Water as needed
- 1 tablespoon chopped almonds, toasted

Directions:

1. Place gelatin in a small bowl and stir in small amount of water according to instructions on the pack, or 1 tablespoon water for 1 teaspoon of gelatin and set aside until bloom.
2. In the meantime, place a small saucepan over medium heat, add remaining ingredients except for almonds, stir well and bring the mixture to a light boil.
3. Then lower heat and simmer mixture for 3 minutes or until mixture begin to thicken.
4. Remove pan from heat, stir in gelatin until dissolved completely and divide the mixture evenly between six ramekins.
5. Cover ramekins with plastic wrap and chill in the refrigerator for 2 hours.
6. When ready to serve, top with toasted almonds and serve.

Nutrition: Calories: 271 Carbs: 2 g Fat: 29 g Protein: 3 g Fiber: 0 g

164. FAT BOMBS

Preparation Time: 15 minutes - Cooking Time: 2 minutes - Servings: 4

Ingredients:

- 1 ½ ounce macadamia nuts halves
- ¼ cup chocolate chips, stevia-sweetened
- 1/8 teaspoon sea salt and more as needed
- 1 tablespoon avocado oil

Directions:

1. Place chocolate chips in a heatproof bowl and microwave for 50 to 60 seconds or until melted.
2. Stir chocolate, and then stir in salt and oil until blended.
3. Take 8 mini muffin cups, place three nuts into each cup and then evenly spoon prepared chocolate mixture, covering nuts completely.
4. Sprinkle with more salt and chill in the freezer for 30 minutes or more until solid.
5. Serve straightaway or store in a plastic bag into the freezer.

Nutrition: Calories: 161 Carbs: 4 g Fat: 16 g Protein: 2 g Fiber: 2 g

165. EASY CHOCOLATE FROSTY

Preparation Time: 10 minutes - Cooking Time: 10 minutes - Servings: 4

Ingredients:

- 1 cup heavy whipping cream - 5 drops liquid stevia - 1 tsp vanilla
- 1 tbsp. almond butter - 2 tbsp. unsweetened cocoa powder

Directions:

1. Add heavy whipping cream into the medium bowl and beat using the hand mixer for 5 minutes. Add remaining ingredients and blend until thick whipped cream form.
2. Pour in serving bowls and place them in the freezer for 30 minutes. Serve and enjoy.

Nutrition: Calories 137 Fat 13.7 g Carbohydrates 3.2 g Sugar 0.4 g Protein 2 g Cholesterol 41 mg

166. EASY BERRY ICE CREAM

Preparation Time: 10 minutes - Cooking Time: 10 minutes - Servings: 6

Ingredients:

- 2/3 cup heavy cream - 2 tbsp. Swerve - 10 oz. frozen berries

Directions:

1. Add frozen berries and Swerve into the food processor and process until just berries are chopped.
2. Add heavy cream and process until smooth. Serve immediately and enjoy it.

Nutrition: Calories 75 Fat 5.1 g Carbohydrates 6.8 g Sugar 3.4 g Protein 0.6 g Cholesterol 18 mg

167. FROZEN WHIPS

Preparation Time: 10 minutes - Cooking Time: 10 minutes - Servings: 12

Ingredients:

- 1 cup heavy whipping cream - 1/2 tsp vanilla - 2 1/2 tbsp. Swerve
- 4 tbsp. unsweetened cocoa powder - Pinch of salt

Directions:

1. Line baking sheet with parchment paper and set aside.
2. Add heavy whipping cream into the large mixing bowl.
3. Add remaining ingredients and stir well.
4. Using a hand mixer beat heavy cream mixture until firm peaks form.
5. Transfer cream mixture into the piping bag. On the prepared baking sheet swirl the cream around into large mounds. Make 12 cream mounds.
6. Place the baking sheet in the freezer for 1 hour. Serve and enjoy.

Nutrition: Calories 40 Fat 4 g Carbohydrates 1.7 g Sugar 0.1 g Protein 0.6 g Cholesterol 14 mg

168. CHOCOLATE ICE CREAM

Preparation Time: 10 minutes - Cooking Time: 10 minutes - Servings: 4

Ingredients:

- 1 cup heavy cream - 2 tbsp. unsweetened chocolate chips - 1 tsp vanilla
- 1 tbsp. unsweetened cocoa powder - 2 tbsp. erythritol

Directions:

1. Add all ingredients into the Mason jar and seal jar with a lid. Shake jar continuously for 5 minutes and place it in the freezer for 6-10 hours. Serve chilled and enjoy.

Nutrition: Calories 160 Fat 15.3 g Carbohydrates 3.7 g Sugar 0.2 g Protein 1.9 g Cholesterol 41 mg

169. NO CHURN ICE CREAM

Preparation Time: 10 minutes - Cooking Time: 10 minutes - Servings: 10

Ingredients:

- 1 1/2 cups heavy cream - 12 oz. strawberries - 1/3 cup Swerve
- 1 tsp vanilla - 1 1/2 cups sour cream - 1/4 cup xylitol

Directions:

1. Add strawberries and xylitol into the blender and blend until pureed.
2. In a mixing bowl, whisk together strawberry mixture, vanilla, and sour cream until well combined. In a separate bowl, beat heavy cream and Swerve until stiff peaks form.
3. Gently fold whipped cream mixture into the strawberry mixture. Transfer in airtight container and place in the refrigerator for 8 hours. Serve and enjoy.

Nutrition: Calories 148 Fat 14 g Carbohydrates 4.7 g Sugar 1.8 g Protein 1.7 g Cholesterol 40 mg

170. CHOCO CHIP ICE CREAM

Preparation Time: 10 minutes - Cooking Time: 10 minutes - Servings: 8

Ingredients:

- 16 oz. heavy whipping cream - 3 oz. unsweetened chocolate chips - 2 tsp vanilla
- 1 cup unsweetened almond milk - 1 tsp peppermint extract - 1/2 cup erythritol

Directions:

1. Add heavy whipping cream into the mixing bowl. Using a hand mixer beat heavy cream until stiff peaks form. Slowly add sweetener and beat well.
2. Add peppermint extract and vanilla and beat for 15 seconds. Slowly add milk and beat well.
3. Pour mixture into the ice cream maker and churn according to the machine instructions.
4. Add chocolate chips at the end and stir well. Transfer mixture into the airtight container and place it in the freezer for 8-10 hours. Serve chilled and enjoy.

Nutrition: Calories 276 Fat 27.1 g Carbohydrates 4.9 g Sugar 0.3 g Protein 2.7 g Cholesterol 78 mg

171. SIMPLE RASPBERRY ICE CREAM

Preparation Time: 5 minutes - Cooking Time: 5 minutes - Servings: 5

Ingredients:

- 2 cups frozen raspberries
- 1 cup heavy cream
- 1/3 cup erythritol

Directions:

1. Add heavy cream into the medium bowl and beat using a hand mixer until stiff peaks form.
2. Add raspberries and sweetener into the blender and blend until pureed.
3. Pour raspberry mixture into the heavy cream and fold well.
4. Serve immediately and enjoy it.

Nutrition: Calories 99 Fat 8.9 g Carbohydrates 4.4 g Sugar 1.9 g Protein 1 g Cholesterol 33 mg

172. CHOCO PEANUT BUTTER ICE CREAM

Preparation Time: 10 minutes - Cooking Time: 10 minutes - Servings: 6

Ingredients:

- 1/2 cup creamy peanut butter
- 1/2 cup Swerve
- 1/4 cup unsweetened cocoa powder
- 1/3 cup coconut oil, melted
- oz. can full-fat coconut milk
- Pinch of salt

Directions:

1. Add all ingredients into the blender and blend until smooth.
2. Pour mixture into the glass container.
3. Cover and place in the freezer for 30 minutes.
4. Stir mixture after 30 minutes, then cover and place in the freezer for 30 minutes.
5. Stir mixture again, then cover and store for 2-3 hours more.
6. Serve chilled and enjoy.

Nutrition: Calories 357 Fat 35.2 g Carbohydrates 8.3 g Sugar 3.1 g Protein 7.1 g Cholesterol 0 mg

173. HEALTHY BLACKBERRY YOGURT

Preparation Time: 5 minutes - Cooking Time: 5 minutes - Servings: 6

Ingredients:

- 4 cups frozen blackberries - 1 tsp vanilla - 1 tbsp. fresh lemon juice - 1 cup Greek yogurt

Directions:

1. Add all ingredients into the blender and blend until smooth.
2. Pour blended mixture into the container and place it in the freezer for 2 hours.
3. Serve and enjoy.

Nutrition: Calories 69 Fat 1.2 g Carbohydrates 10.7 g Sugar 6.2 g Protein 4.7 g Cholesterol 2 mg

174. DELICIOUS FROZEN HOT CHOCOLATE

Preparation Time: 5 minutes Cooking Time: 5 minutes Servings: 1

Ingredients:

- 3 tbsp. heavy cream - 1 tbsp. coconut oil - 1/2 tsp vanilla
- 3 tbsp. unsweetened cocoa powder - 3 tbsp. Swerve
- 1 cup unsweetened almond milk - 1 cup of ice cubes

Directions:

1. Add all ingredients into the blender and blend until smooth.
2. Serve and enjoy.

Nutrition: Calories 272 Fat 24.7 g Carbohydrates 18.1g Sugar 1.6 g Protein 4.7 g Cholesterol 20 mg

175. CREAMY STRAWBERRY YOGURT

Preparation Time: 5 minutes - Cooking Time: 5 minutes - Servings: 8

Ingredients:

- 4 cups frozen strawberries
- 1 tbsp. fresh lemon juice
- 1/4 cup erythritol
- 1/2 cup Greek yogurt

Directions:

1. Add all ingredients into the food processor and process until creamy.
2. Serve immediately and enjoy it.

Nutrition: Calories 39 Fat 0.4 g Carbohydrates 7.3 g Sugar 5.2 g Protein 1.8 g Cholesterol 1 mg

176. SWEET STRAWBERRY POPSICLES

Preparation Time: 10 minutes - Cooking Time: 5 minutes - Servings: 8

Ingredients:

- 1 1/2 cups frozen strawberries, thawed & chopped
- 2 tbsp. Swerve - 1 tsp vanilla
- 1 scoop whey protein powder
- 2 tsp fresh lime juice - 1 cup heavy cream

Directions:

1. Add heavy cream in a large bowl and beat using a hand mixer until soft peaks form.
2. Add remaining ingredients and fold gently.
3. Spoon heavy cream mixture into the popsicle molds and place in the freezer for 1 hour or until firm.
4. Serve and enjoy.

Nutrition: Calories 79 Fat 5.8 g Carbohydrates 4 g Sugar 1.9 g Protein 3.1 g Cholesterol 29 mg

177. FROZEN STRAWBERRY CUPCAKES

Preparation Time: 10 minutes - Cooking Time: 10 minutes - Servings: 6

Ingredients:

- 1 cup strawberries
- 1 cup greek yogurt
- 3 tbsp. erythritol
- 2 tbsp. butter, melted
- 1/3 cup almond flour

Directions:

1. Line 6-cups muffin tray with cupcake liners and set aside.
2. In a medium bowl, mix together almond flour, half sweetener, and butter.
3. Divide the almond flour mixture into the muffin cups and press down slightly.
4. Add half strawberries, yogurt, and remaining sweetener into the blender and blend until smooth.
5. Spoon strawberry mixture into the muffin cups.
6. Cut remaining strawberries into the slices. Place strawberry slices on top of each cupcake.
7. Place the cupcake in the freezer for 6 hours or until firm.
8. Serve and enjoy.

Nutrition: Calories 115 Fat 7.8 g Carbohydrates 5.1 g Sugar 3.1 g Protein 6.3 g Cholesterol 13 mg

178. LEMON ICE CREAM

Preparation Time: 5 minutes - Cooking Time: 5 minutes - Servings: 8

Ingredients:

- 4 egg yolks
- 1/2 cup fresh lemon juice
- 1 tsp liquid stevia
- 2 tsp lemon zest
- 4 cups full-fat coconut milk
- Pinch of salt

Directions:

1. Add all ingredients into the blender and blend until smooth.
2. Pour mixture into the ice cream maker and churn according to the machine instructions.
3. Pour into the airtight container and place it in the freezer until set.
4. Serve chilled and enjoy.

Nutrition: Calories 86 Fat 7.9 g Carbohydrates 1.2 g Sugar 0.4 g Protein 2 g Cholesterol 105 mg

179. EASY BLACKBERRY GELATO

Preparation Time: 10 minutes - Cooking Time: 10 minutes - Servings: 8

Ingredients:

- 8 oz. frozen blackberries
- 1 tbsp. MCT oil
- 1/2 tsp liquid stevia
- 4 oz. Swerve
- 8 oz. heavy cream
- 12 oz. unsweetened almond milk
- Pinch of salt

Directions:

1. Add all ingredients into the blender and blend until smooth.
2. Pour mixture into the ice cream maker and churn according to the machine instructions.
3. Pour into the loaf pan and place it in the freezer for 3 hours.
4. Serve chilled and enjoy.

Nutrition: Calories 132 Fat 13 g Carbohydrates 4.9 g Sugar 1.4 g Protein 1.1 g Cholesterol 39 mg

180. QUICK RASPBERRY ICE CREAM

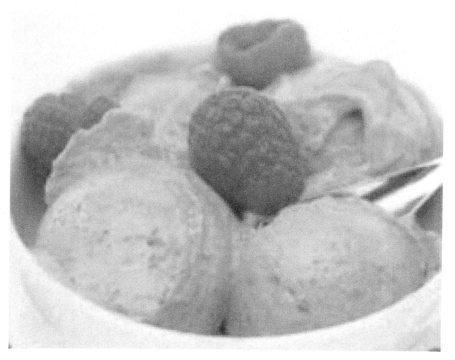

Preparation Time: 5 minutes - Cooking Time: 5 minutes - Servings: 2

Ingredients:

- 1 cup frozen raspberries
- 1/8 tsp stevia powder
- 1/2 cup heavy cream

Directions:

1. Add all ingredients into the food processor and process until smooth.
2. Serve immediately and enjoy it.

Nutrition: Calories 144 Fat 11.1 g Carbohydrates 10.2 g Sugar 4.7 g Protein 2 g Cholesterol 41 mg

BROWNIE RECIPES

181. CHOCOLATE BROWNIES

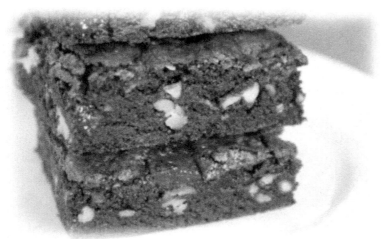

Preparation Time: 10 minutes - Cooking Time: 25 minutes - Servings: 6

Ingredients:

- 3 large eggs - 1/4 cup unsweetened cocoa powder - 2 tbsp. butter, melted
- 1/4 cup flaxseed meal - 3/4 cup almond flour - 2 tsp vanilla
- 2 tsp baking powder - 1/4 cup Swerve - 1/4 cup almonds, chopped - 1/3 cup coconut cream

Directions:

1. In a large bowl, mix together the almond flour, baking powder, swerve, cocoa powder, and flaxseed meal.
2. Add the eggs, coconut cream, almond, vanilla, and butter.
3. Beat using a blender until well combined. Spray a baking dish with cooking spray.
4. Pour batter into the prepared dish and cover with foil. Set aside.
5. Pour 2 cups of water into the instant pot then place a trivet in the pot.
6. Place baking dish on top of the trivet.
7. Seal pot with lid and cook on high for 25 minutes.
8. Release pressure using quick release method then open the lid.
9. Cut into the slices and serve.

Nutrition: Calories 242 Fat 20.5 g Carbohydrates 9 g Sugar 1.6 g Protein 8.9 g Cholesterol 103 mg

182. DELICIOUS HAZELNUTS BROWNIES

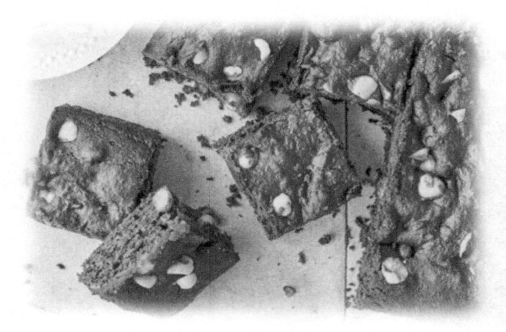

Preparation Time: 10 minutes - Cooking Time: 25 minutes - Servings: 6

Ingredients:

- 4 eggs - 1 tsp vanilla - 1/4 cup hazelnuts, chopped - 1/4 cup Swerve
- 3/4 cup almond flour - 1/4 cup unsweetened cocoa powder - 2 tbsp. butter
- 1/2 cup mascarpone - 1/2 cup flaxseed meal - Pinch of salt

Directions:

1. In a large bowl, add all ingredients except hazelnuts and beat until smooth.
2. Add hazelnuts fold well.
3. Grease baking dish with butter and line with parchment paper.
4. Pour batter into the prepared dish.
5. Pour 1 cup of water into the instant pot then place a trivet in the pot.
6. Place dish on top of the trivet.
7. Seal pot with lid and cook on high for 25 minutes.
8. Release pressure using quick release method then open the lid.
9. Cut into pieces and serve.

Nutrition: Calories 263 Fat 21.3 g Carbohydrates 7.2g Sugar 1.2g Protein 11.3 g Cholesterol 130 mg

183. CINNAMON BERRY BROWNIES

Preparation Time: 10 minutes - Cooking Time: 3 minutes - Servings: 6

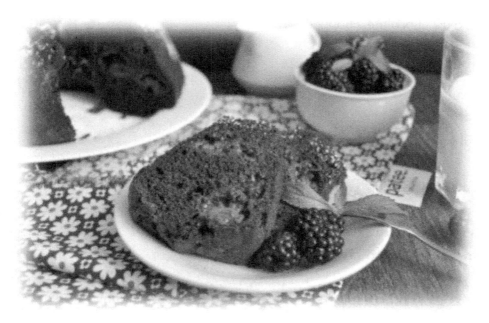

Ingredients:

- 1/4 cup almond butter - 1/4 tsp cinnamon - 3 tbsp. swerve
- 1/4 cup yogurt - 1/4 cup coconut flour - 1/4 cup fresh blackberries
- 1/4 cup coconut oil - ¼ cup unsweetened cocoa powder

Directions:

1. Spray a baking dish with cooking spray and set aside.
2. Pour 1 cup of water into the instant pot then place a trivet in the pot.
3. Add all ingredients into a large bowl and beat using a hand mixer for 2-3 minutes.
4. Pour batter into the prepared baking dish.
5. Place dish on top of the trivet.
6. Seal pot with lid and cook on high for 3 minutes.
7. Allow to release pressure naturally then open the lid.
8. Serve and enjoy.

Nutrition: Calories 97 Fat 9.7 g Carbohydrates 2.8 g Sugar 1.1 g Protein 0.9 g Cholesterol 1 mg

184. FUDGY MUG BROWNIE

Preparation Time: 5 minutes - Cooking Time: 1 minute - Servings: 1

Ingredients:

- 1 tbsp. unsweetened dark chocolate, chopped
- 1 tsp olive oil
- 1 1/2 tbsp. water
- 1 1/2 tbsp. heavy cream
- 1 1/2 tbsp. Swerve
- 1/2 tsp baking powder
- 2 tsp coconut flour
- 2 tbsp. unsweetened cocoa powder

Directions:

1. Add all ingredients into the microwave-safe mug and mix until smooth.
2. Place mug in microwave and microwave for 1 minute.
3. Serve and enjoy.

Nutrition: Calories 228 Fat 21 g Carbohydrates 16.8 g Sugar 0.2 g Protein 4.9 g Cholesterol 31 mg

185. PEANUT BUTTER BROWNIES

Preparation Time: 5 minutes - Cooking Time: 15 minutes - Servings: 12

Ingredients:

- 2 eggs -2 tbsp. peanut butter - 1 tsp vanilla
- 1/4 cup unsweetened cocoa powder
- 1/2 cup butter, melted - 1/4 cup Swerve
- 3/4 cup almond flour - Pinch of salt

Directions:

1. Preheat the oven to 450 F.
2. Line 8*8-inch baking pan with parchment paper and set aside.
3. In a large bowl, mix together almond flour and sweetener.
4. Add remaining ingredients into the almond flour mixture and mix until well combined.
5. Pour batter into the prepared pan and bake for 15 minutes.
6. Slice and serve.

Nutrition: Calories 144 Fat 13.7 g Carbohydrates 2.9 g Sugar 0.6 g Protein 2 g Cholesterol 48 mg

186. CHOCO CHIP MUG BROWNIE

Preparation Time: 5 minutes - Cooking Time: 1 minute - Servings: 1

Ingredients:

- 2 tbsp. unsweetened almond milk
- 1/4 tsp vanilla
- 1 tbsp. unsweetened cocoa powder
- 2 tbsp. Swerve
- 1/3 cup almond flour
- 2 tbsp. unsweetened chocolate chips
- 1 tbsp. butter, melted
- Pinch of salt

Directions:

1. Add all ingredients except chocolate chips into the microwave-safe mug and mix until smooth.
2. Add chocolate chips and stir well.
3. Place mug in microwave and microwave for 1 minute.
4. Serve and enjoy.

Nutrition: Calories 163 Fat 14.5 g Carbohydrates 10.4 g Sugar 2.5 g Protein 1.5 g Cholesterol 31 mg

187. FLOURLESS BROWNIES

Preparation Time: 10 minutes - Cooking Time: 20 minutes - Servings: 12

Ingredients:

- 6 eggs - 4 tbsp. Swerve
- 4 oz. cream cheese, softened
- 2 tsp vanilla - 1/2 tsp baking powder
- 2/3 cup unsweetened cocoa powder
- 1 1/2 sticks butter, melted

Directions:

1. Add all ingredients into the mixing bowl and beat until smooth using a hand mixer.
2. Pour mixture into the greased square baking dish and bake at 350 F for 20-25 minutes.
3. Slice and serve.

Nutrition: Calories 181 Fat 17.6 g Carbohydrates 4 g Sugar 0.4 g Protein 4.5 g Cholesterol 123 mg

188. PROTEIN BROWNIE

Preparation Time: 10 minutes - Cooking Time: 15 minutes - Servings: 8

Ingredients:

- 2 scoops chocolate protein powder
- 1/2 tsp vanilla
- 3 tbsp. coconut butter, melted
- 4 egg whites - 1/4 tsp salt
- 3 tbsp. unsweetened cocoa powder
- 1/4 cup Swerve
- 1/4 cup almond flour

Directions:

1. Preheat the oven to 300 F.
2. Grease 7*5-inch baking dish and set aside.
3. In a medium bowl, mix together dry ingredients.
4. Add egg whites, vanilla, and melted coconut butter into the mixing bowl and beat until smooth.
5. Add dry mixture into the egg white mixture and mix until well combined.
6. Pour batter into the prepared pan and bake for 15 minutes.
7. Slice and serve.

Nutrition: Calories 63 Fat 3.6 g Carbohydrates 2.9 g Sugar 0.7 g Protein 4.8 g Cholesterol 5 mg

189. DELICIOUS BROWNIE BITES

Preparation Time: 10 minutes - Cooking Time: 20 minutes - Servings: 12

Ingredients:

- 6 eggs - 1/2 cup walnuts, chopped
- 4 tbsp. Swerve - oz. cream cheese
- 2 tsp vanilla - 1/2 tsp baking powder
- 2.2 oz. unsweetened cocoa powder - oz. butter, melted

Directions:

1. Add all ingredients except walnuts into the mixing bowl and beat until smooth.
2. Add walnuts and stir well.
3. Pour batter into the greased baking dish and bake for 20-25 minutes at 350 F.
4. Slice and serve.

Nutrition: Calories 209 Fat 20.2 g Carbohydrates 4.6 g Sugar 0.4 g Protein 6 g Cholesterol 121 mg

190. ZUCCHINI NUT-FREE BROWNIES

Preparation Time: 10 minutes - Cooking Time: 20 minutes - Servings: 6

Ingredients:

- 2 eggs, lightly beaten
- 1/2 cup unsweetened cocoa powder
- 1/4 cup unsweetened coconut milk
- 1/4 cup Swerve
- 1 cup sun butter
- 1 medium zucchini, shredded and squeeze out all liquid
- 1/4 cup coconut flour

Directions:

1. Preheat the oven to 350 F.
2. Line 8*8-inch baking dish with parchment paper and set aside.
3. In a large bowl, mix together sun butter, milk, and eggs.
4. Add coconut flour, sweetener, zucchini, and cocoa powder and stir to combine.
5. Transfer mixture in prepare dish and bake for 20 minutes.
6. Slice and serve.

Nutrition: Calories 161 Fat 9.1 g Carbohydrates 17.9 g Sugar 6.6 g Protein 6.1 g Cholesterol 55 mg

191. COCOA ALMOND BUTTER BROWNIES

Preparation Time: 10 minutes - Cooking Time: 20 minutes - Servings: 4

Ingredients:

- 1/2 cup almond butter, melted
- 1 cup bananas, overripe
- 1 scoop whey protein powder
- 2 tbsp. unsweetened cocoa powder
- 2 tbsp. walnuts, chopped

Directions:

1. Preheat the oven to 350 F. Spray brownie tray with cooking spray.
2. Add all ingredients except walnut into the blender and blend until smooth.
3. Pour batter into the prepared dish. Add walnuts into the batter and mix well and bake for 20 minutes.
4. Serve and enjoy.

Nutrition: Calories 106 Fat 4.4 g Carbohydrates 11.7 g Sugar 5 g Protein 7.9 g Cholesterol 16 mg

192. PROTEIN MUG BROWNIE

Preparation Time: 10 minutes - Cooking Time: 1 minute - Servings: 1

Ingredients:

- 1 scoop chocolate protein powder
- 1/2 tsp baking powder
- 1/4 cup almond milk
- 1 tbsp. cocoa powder

Directions:

1. In a microwave-safe mug mix together baking powder, protein powder, and cocoa.
2. Add almond milk and stir well.
3. Place mug in microwave and microwave for 30 seconds.
4. Serve and enjoy.

Nutrition: Calories 207 Fat 15.8 g Carbohydrates 9.5 g Sugar 3 g Protein 12.4 g Cholesterol 20 mg

193. AVOCADO BROWNIES

Preparation Time: 10 minutes - Cooking Time: 35 minutes - Servings: 9

Ingredients:

- 2 eggs
- 1 tsp baking powder
- 2 tbsp. swerve
- 2 avocados, mashed
- 1/3 cup chocolate chips, melted
- 4 tbsp. coconut oil, melted
- 2/3 cup unsweetened cocoa powder

Directions:

1. Preheat the oven to 325 F.
2. In a large bowl, mix together all dry ingredients.
3. In another bowl, mix together avocado and eggs until well combined.
4. Slowly add dry mixture to the wet along with melted chocolate and oil. Mix well.
5. Pour batter in a greased baking pan and bake for 30-35 minutes.
6. Slice and serve.

Nutrition: Calories 207 Fat 18 g Carbohydrates 11 g Sugar 3.6 g Protein 3.8 g Cholesterol 38 mg

194. EASY MUG BROWNIE

Preparation Time: 10 minutes - Cooking Time: 1 minute - Servings: 1

Ingredients:

- 2 eggs
- 1 tbsp. erythritol
- 1/4 tsp vanilla
- 1 tbsp. heavy cream
- 1 scoop protein powder

Directions:

1. Add all ingredients into the mug and mix well.
2. Place mug in microwave and microwave for 1 minute.
3. Serve and enjoy.

Nutrition: Calories 305 Fat 16 g Carbohydrates 7 g Sugar 1.8 g Protein 33 g Cholesterol 412 mg

195. CHOCOLATE BANANA BROWNIE

Preparation Time: 10 minutes - Cooking Time: 16 minutes - Servings: 4

Ingredients:

- 1 scoop protein powder
- 2 tbsp. unsweetened cocoa powder
- 1 cup bananas, overripe
- 1/2 cup almond butter, melted

Directions:

1. Preheat the air fryer to 325 F.
2. Spray air fryer baking pan with cooking spray.
3. Add all ingredients into the blender and blend until smooth.
4. Pour batter into the prepared pan and place in the air fryer basket and cook brownie for 16 minutes.
5. Serve and enjoy.

Nutrition: Calories 82 Fat 2.1 g Carbohydrates 11.3 g Sugar 5 g Protein 6.9 g Cholesterol 16 mg

196. DELICIOUS FUDGY BROWNIES

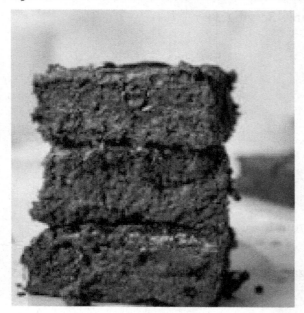

Preparation Time: 10 minutes - Cooking Time: 16 minutes - Servings: 6

Ingredients:

- 3 eggs - 1/2 tsp baking powder
- 3/4 cup erythritol
- 2 oz. unsweetened dark chocolate
- 3/4 cup butter softened
- 1/2 cup almond flour
- 1/4 cup unsweetened cocoa powder

Directions:

1. Preheat the air fryer to 325 F. Spray air fryer baking dish with cooking spray and set aside.
2. In a bowl, mix together chocolate and butter and microwave for 30 seconds or until melted. Stir well.
3. Mix together almond flour, baking powder, cocoa powder, and sweetener.
4. In a mixing bowl beat eggs using a hand mixer. Add the chocolate-butter mixture and beat until combined.
5. Slowly add dry ingredients and mix until combined.
6. Pour batter into the prepared dish and place it into the air fryer and cook for 16 minutes.
7. Slice and serve.

Nutrition: Calories 367 Fat 35.7 g Carbohydrates 6.5 g Sugar 0.6 g Protein 5 g Cholesterol 143 mg

197. MOLTEN BROWNIE CUPS

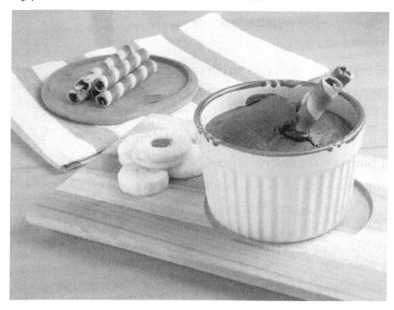

Preparation Time: 10 minutes - Cooking Time: 9 minutes - Servings: 4

Ingredients:

- Chocolate chips, sugar-free – 2/3 cup; Butter, salted – 6 tablespoons
- Eggs – 3; Swerve sweetener – 2/3 cup; Almond flour – 3 ½ tablespoons
- Vanilla extract, unsweetened – 1 teaspoon; Water – 1 3/4 cups

Directions:

1. Take a medium saucepan, place it over medium-low heat, add chocolate chips and butter and cook for 5 minutes or until chocolate and butter melts and is blended, stirring frequently.

2. Crack eggs in a bowl, add flour, sweetener, and vanilla, whisk until blended, and then whisk in chocolate mixture until combined.

3. Take four 6-ounce ramekins, grease them with avocado oil and then evenly pour in muffin batter until halfway full. Switch on the instant pot, pour in water, then insert a trivet stand and stack ramekins on it.

4. Shut the instant pot with its lid in the sealed position, then press the 'manual' button, press '+/-' to set the cooking time to 9 minutes and cook at high-pressure setting; when the pressure builds in the pot, the cooking timer will start.

5. When the instant pot buzzes, press the 'keep warm' button, do a quick pressure release and open the lid.

6. Take out the ramekins, let cool for 10 minutes at room temperature, then garnish with cream and serve.

Nutrition: Calories 425 Fat 36 g Protein 9 g Net Carbs 7 g Fiber 3 g

198. INCREDIBLY FUDGY BROWNIES

Preparation time: 15 minutes - Cooking time: 15 – 20 minutes - Servings: 16

Ingredients:

- 9 tbsp. butter - 2/3 cup powdered erythritol - 3/4 cup almond flour
- 11 tbsp. unsweetened cocoa powder - 3 eggs, room temperature - 1/2 tsp. kosher salt

Directions:

1. Preheat oven to 350 degrees F. Put water in a small pot to a gentle simmer.
2. In a heat-proof mixing bowl, combine cocoa powder, butter, salt, and sweetener.
3. Put bowl on top of the pot of simmering water and whisk until the sweetener has dissolved.
4. Allow the mixture to cool. Add eggs, whisking until incorporated before adding the succeeding one. Whisk until smooth.
5. Whisk in the almond flour. Stop whisking when you can no longer see lumps of flour. Don't over mix or your brownies will come out cakey and tough rather than fudgy.
6. Pour into a lined pan. Bake for around 15 to 25 minutes or until the center is just set, with a slight jiggle. If you want fudgier brownies, take your brownies out of the oven before the batter has fully set, when it is slightly under baked.
7. Take out the pan and cool on a rack. Cut into 16 squares.

Nutrition:Calories: 102 Fat: 9 g Carbohydrates: 1 g Protein: 2 g

199. BROWNIE BALLS

Preparation time: 20 minutes - Cooking time: 14 – 18 minutes - Servings: 16

Ingredients:

- 4 tbsp. butter - 1/2 cup unsweetened cocoa powder - 3/4 cup monk fruit sweetener
- 3/4 cup super fine almond flour - 2 eggs - 1/4 tsp. kosher salt
- 1/4 cup walnuts, chopped - 1/2 tsp. vanilla extract

Directions:

1. Start to preheat oven to 350 degrees F. In a large mixing bowl, combine butter, cocoa powder, sweetener, vanilla extract, eggs, and salt. Whisk until well combined.
2. Stir in almond flour and walnuts and mix using spatula. Don't over mix.
3. Scoop the brownie mixture into the wells of a mini silicone muffin pan.
4. Put the pan on top of a sturdier baking tray. Place the tray and muffin pan in the center of the oven.
5. Bake for 14 to 18 minutes. If you want fudgy brownies, bake for around 14-16. If you want cakey brownies, go for 17-18.
6. Cool brownies on rack.

Nutrition: Calories: 69 Fat: 6 g Carbohydrates: 2 g Protein: 2 g

200. CHEESECAKE BROWNIES

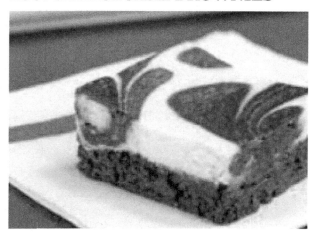

Preparation time: 25 minutes - Cooking time: 15 – 25 minutes - Servings: 16

Ingredients:

For the brownie:

- 9 tbsp. butter - 2/3 cup powdered erythritol - 3/4 cup almond flour
- 11 tbsp. unsweetened cocoa powder - 3 eggs - 1/2 tsp. kosher salt

For the cheesecake:

- 8 oz. cream cheese - 1 egg - 1/4 cup erythritol - 1 tsp. vanilla extract

Directions:

1. Start to preheat oven to 350 degrees F. Line the sides and bottom of an 8x8-inch baking pan with parchment paper. Set aside.
2. First make the cheesecake layer. In a bowl, combine cream cheese with your sweetener and cream until smooth. Add vanilla extract and the egg. Whisk until well incorporated. Set aside.
3. Do the brownie layer. Put water in a small pot to a gentle simmer. In a heat-proof mixing bowl, combine cocoa powder, butter, salt, and sweetener. Put bowl on top of the pot of simmering water and whisk until the sweetener has dissolved.
4. Allow the mixture to cool. Add eggs while whisking until incorporated before adding the succeeding one. Whisk until smooth.
5. Whisk in the almond flour. Stop whisking when you can no longer see lumps of flour. Don't over mix or your brownies will come out cakey and tough rather than fudgy.
6. Pour 2/3 of the brownie batter into lined pan. Pour in the cheesecake batter. Pour the last 1/3 of the brownie batter in four separate dollops and swirl the two mixtures using a toothpick or a knife to create a nice marbled effect.
7. Bake for 15 to 25 minutes or until the center is just set, with a slight jiggle.
8. Take out the pan and cool on a rack. Cut into 16 squares.

Nutrition: Calories: 155 Fat: 15 g Carbohydrates: 1.5 g Protein: 4 g

CONCLUSION

When you're looking to start a keto diet, making the right food choices can be difficult. What seems like a small portion of food can end up being much larger than anticipated. As a result, many people struggle to stay within their calorie limits on their keto diet.

If you're struggling to stay within your daily calorie budget on keto, we have the perfect solution for you.

When you are on a ketogenic diet, it is important to ensure that you don't overindulge in food. That's why we have put together a keto dessert cookbook that will give you the ultimate variety of delicious recipes that are keto-friendly!

In addition to having a wide range of desserts, this book also features a wide range of other delicious recipes that you can add to your diet. It has recipes for everything from easy breakfasts to mouthwatering main dishes and even more!

Whether you are going on a keto diet or not, this book is great for anyone who loves to cook. It provides all the information that you need so that you can start cooking meals that will leave you feeling full and satisfied. Besides giving you an array of recipes, this book also helps you understand how different types of foods work together so that you can have great tasting meals whether you are on a keto diet or not.

Keto diet is an eating plan that is low in carbohydrates and high in fats. The goal of the keto diet is to put your body into a metabolic state called "ketosis", which occurs when the body burns fat instead of carbs for energy. The result is that your body starts using fat and protein as fuel instead of glucose, which means you lose weight.

People on the keto diet may eat as much fat and protein as they want, but it's important to eat sources of healthy fats and healthy protein. In fact, most keto dieters choose lean proteins like fish, chicken, beef, pork and eggs over red meats and full-fat dairy products. Because a portion of your daily calories on the keto diet must come from fat (including saturated fat), it's important to include some fat in your keto meal plan – even if it's just a source of healthy monounsaturated or polyunsaturated Fat like olive oil or fish oil.

We have compiled a list of the best keto desserts available in this book! This list is by no means comprehensive, but it is a great place to start. We hope this helps you find a keto friendly dessert that is new to your taste buds! If you think we have missed any great keto desserts, please let us know and we will add them to our list.

Made in the USA
Middletown, DE
06 November 2021